NATURAL THERAPEUTICS

Volume 3

NATURAL DIETETICS

HENRY LINDLAHR, M.D.

EDITED AND REVISED BY

JOCELYN C. P. PROBY
M.A., M.Litt(Oxon), D.O.(Kirksville, U.S.A.)

SAFFRON WALDEN
THE C. W. DANIEL COMPANY LIMITED

First published in this edition by
The C. W. Daniel Company Limited
1 Church Path, Saffron Walden, Essex CB10 1JP, England

ISBN 0 85207 155 8

.

Set in Great Britain by the White Crescent Press Ltd, Luton, Beds
and printed and bound by Hillman Printers, Frome, Somerset

CONTENTS

		Page
Editor's Introduction		v
Preface		xi
I.	Why We Favour a Vegetarian Diet	1
II.	Is it Worth While to Pay Attention to Diet?	6
III.	For What do We Eat and Drink?	11
IV.	The Normal Functions of Food and Drink in the Economy	18
V.	The Destructive Effects of Food and Drink	24
VI.	The Tensing and Relaxing Effects of Foods Upon the Digestive Organs and the System as a Whole	28
VII.	Standard Foods	32
VIII.	Digestion and Assimilation	36
IX.	The True Nature and Source of Vitamins or Life Elements	40
X.	Who Discovered the Vitamins or Life Elements?	45
XI.	What are the Life Elements?	50
XII.	Relationship of Mineral Salts to Vitamins	53
XIII.	The Fallacy of the Calorie	56
XIV.	Vitamins or Life Elements	64
XV.	How to Charge Foods with Mineral Elements and Vitamins	69

XVI.	Questions and Answers Concerning Vitamins	73
XVII.	The Magnetic Properties of Food	76
XVIII.	Classification of Foods According to Their Mineral Contents and Vitamin Values	82
	Editor's Foreword to Chapter XVIII.	82
XIX.	Miscellaneous	94

Appendices

I.	Key to Our System of Recipe Marking	111
II.	Uncooked Food Versus Cooked Food	117
III.	Medicinal Vegetables and Recipes	123
IV.	Popular Superstitions	126
V.	Classification of Recipes	128
VI.	Some Sample Recipes and Menus	148

Reference Index	163

EDITOR'S INTRODUCTION

Lindlahr's third volume is entitled "The Lindlahr Vegetarian Cook Book and A B C of Natural Dietetics". As the title implies, the book has two parts and in bringing out a new edition I have decided that the Cook Book section should not be included as a whole for several reasons. First, there are now many good vegetarian and other cook books in circulation, secondly, the Lindlahr book is, perhaps, more suited to American tastes and conditions than to English or European, and thirdly, it seems to be in some respects somewhat out of date for use by the average modern housewife. There are, however, many things in the Cook Book section which are extremely valuable as giving much help to persons wishing to follow in practice the kind of diet which is advocated in the "ABC" section of the book. In particular, the way in which Lindlahr classified foods and recipes according to their chemical composition and nutritional function is of great interest and importance. This was intended to assist patients and their wives, nurses and doctors to devise meals and regimens which were well balanced and conformed to the principles which he laid down, both in health and in disease. Accordingly I have added appendices giving extracts from the Cook Book section and a certain number of sample menus and recipes in order to give help and guidance to those seeking to conform to the principles of Natural Dietetics. With the help of the Key in Appendix I and the Analysis Chart in Chapter XVIII it should be possible for anyone wishing to do so to mark the recipes in any Cook Book which he uses so that he can see at a glance the classification to which each recipe belongs.

However, far the most important part of the book is the A B C of Natural Dietetics which is very full and clear and, in parts, very original and revolutionary. A number of points are worthy of special note.

(1) Lindlahr lays great emphasis on the fact that health begins in the soil. This idea has very much come to the fore in recent years under the influence of pioneers of the movement for organic agriculture such as Sir Albert Howard and such organizations as the Soil Association, but Lindlahr lived slightly before this time. He appears to have derived his ideas largely from Julius Hensel, and his description of the methods

which he used in growing produce for himself and for the sanatorium which he founded is of great interest. His form of organic agriculture laid special emphasis on the importance of maintaining the positive mineral content of the soil as well as the level of humus derived from animal and vegetable residues.

(2) Lindlahr's most revolutionary idea is his complete rejection of the caloric theory of diet by which the value of foods is judged almost entirely by the number of calories which they contain. According to him, and he develops his arguments very convincingly, man must not be looked upon as a sort of internal combustion engine into which you put fuel and get out energy and heat. The body does indeed require a certain amount of fuel material which assists it to produce heat and muscular energy, but this is not the only or the primary purpose of food. The human body is a physical and chemical organization in which various forms of energy are functioning and the main purpose of food is to provide material for the building and repair of tissues and to maintain a proper chemical and fluid balance in the body so that the processes of absorption and elimination can take place in a satisfactory manner. Sound dietetics is largely a matter of proportion and balance and requires a knowledge of the chemical composition of various foods such as is supplied by the various charts and tables which he gives.

(3) Lindlahr is not an advocate of the high protein diets which are considered desirable by so many nutritionists. A certain amount of protein is necessary and desirable, especially in youth, for the building up and repair of tissues, but the high protein foods are acid forming and are only required in very limited quantities. It is noteworthy that milk which is the natural food of the youngest humans and animals when they are growing fast is not what is considered a high protein food. It is also noteworthy that the animals which are generally eaten to provide protein meals live entirely on what is generally regarded as a low protein diet.

(4) Lindlahr looks upon man as being naturally a vegetarian or fruitarian animal. On the basis of comparative anatomy he is allied to vegetarian and frugivirous, rather than carnivorous, animals. Moreover, as most foods are rendered less nutritious by cooking, a large proportion of what we eat should be eaten raw. There are, of course, many arguments in favour of vegetarianism and Lindlahr goes into these at some length, though more has been written on the subject since his time. His disciple, Daniel Mackinnon, when discussing the subject was wont to go back to the legend of Prometheus and to Shelley's notes which accompany his poem "Queen Mab". More recently an interesting book entitled "The Recovery of Culture" by Henry Bailey Stevens

seems to throw some light on how early man may have deserted his original vegetarian or garden culture and become first a hunter and a fisherman and later developed cultures based more and more on animal husbandry. At the present time more and more people are coming to realise that, apart from humanitarian considerations, there is much evidence that meat eating is responsible for much disease and that the kind of use of the land to which it gives rise is extremely wasteful of the available land resources even when it does not promote soil erosion and the making of deserts. Lindlahr does not, however, rule out the use of meat entirely in all circumstances and he points out that there are good and bad forms of vegetarianism and hints that the latter may be worse than a good mixed diet containing a certain amount of meat. He is also very strongly in favour of the inclusion in the dietary of the dairy products, eggs and honey because they contain the animal life element and can be taken with little or no cooking. He also states that fish, and especially sea fish, can be very rich in positive mineral elements and may be a useful source of vitamins.

(5) Since Lindlahr's time a great deal of study and research has been devoted to vitamins and amino-acids. What he says on these topics would seem to be sound enough as far as it goes, but I have inserted notes drawing attention to the fact that somewhat more is known on these subjects than in his time, though this would seem to confirm rather than to invalidate what he has to say. A point of interest is that there seems to be a connection between the vitamins and the positive mineral elements in food though they are not exactly the same. Vitamins are chemical entities but they are something more, being in a definite way living and thus liable to destruction by heating and in other ways. This has a bearing on the use of vitamin preparations in cases where a vitamin deficiency is diagnosed, or when the diet is obviously very deficient in vitamins. Lindlahr is not alone in the opinion that synthetic vitamins made in a laboratory are to be avoided and can be harmful as well as ineffective. There are, however, vitamin preparations made from natural sources which can be very useful. In the case of mineral deficiency a similar controversy has arisen as to how far mineral deficiencies such as of sodium, iron, potassium, etc., can or should be made up by inorganic preparations. Lindlahr was of the opinion that such preparations should not be used with the possible exception of small quantities of common salt. On the other hand, there is a school of biochemic therapy which maintains that there is no difference between "organic" and "inorganic" minerals and that the body is able to use inorganic minerals satisfactorily and without harm if they are properly ground down, triturated and prepared. Lindlahr's

great criterion for deciding whether a medicinal preparation was good or bad was to observe whether iridiagnosis revealed its retention in the tissues as is the case, for instance, where iron tonics have been used. Basically I would feel that Lindlahr's way of looking at the matter is the right one and that vitamin and mineral deficiencies should be made up by a change in diet and by the use of such things as fruit and vegetable juices. On the other hand, there may be an argument in favour of the use of some of the biochemic supplementals in an emergency or as a temporary measure. It must also be remembered that many deficiencies as, for instance, of iron, are due not so much to a deficiency in the diet as to a failure in metabolism which may require to be dealt with in another way. Some such conditions, it would appear, are susceptible to homoeopathic treatment.

(6) The tables and charts with Lindlahr gives in various parts of the book and particularly in the Food Analysis Chart are of great value and interest. Some of these could probably be developed, revised and enlarged. The Food Analysis Chart, for instance, would seem to point the way to a means by which the quality of foods could be scientifically tested and recorded and correlated to the condition of the soil and the methods of cultivation and fertilization used in their production. Everyone with experience knows that fruits and vegetables grown on sound organic lines are superior in taste and flavour, in disease resistance and in keeping quality to produce grown in other ways, but it would be good if this superiority could be given support and corroboration by chemical analysis. This appears to have been done in the Analysis Chart in the case of potatoes, but the same thing could doubtless be done for some or all of the other common field and garden crops.

ACKNOWLEDGEMENTS

I wish to express my thanks to the many friends who have helped me in the preparation of this volume, by giving advice and information and by typing and reading proofs. I would like to make special mention of Dr Elizabeth Ogden, Dr J. L. Mount, Dr Douglas Latto, Mrs Veronica Phillips and Mrs J. G. S. Lawson.

Jocelyn Proby, Warmington, Peterborough, 1983

PREFACE

This volume on the subject of Natural Dietetics represents a revised edition of the *Nature Cure Cook Book* first published in 1914. Revision and enlargement became a necessity for several reasons. Since the first edition of the *Nature Cure Cook Book* was published, many new and highly important discoveries have been made in the field of food chemistry and scientific dietetics. Outstanding among these are the discoveries of the Amino-acids and of the Vitamins. It is a remarkable fact that these epoch-making revelations of modern up-to-date science confirm many of the fundamental teachings of *Nature Cure Philosophy and Practice* and of *The Lindlahr System of Natural Dietetics*, which only a few years ago were condemned and ridiculed by orthodox science as visionary theories of ignorant tyros and faddists.

Strict vegetarians and advocates of unfired food criticized our *Nature Cure Cook Book* for containing spices, condiments, combinations too rich in starch and protein and too many cooked food recipes. Those who prefer to live on uncooked food can find hundreds of raw food recipes and useful suggestions for the selection and combination of unfired food. But this book is not intended for those alone who have already solved their dietetic problems. A person living on raw food does not need a cook book, but those who have adopted the Edenic way of living are still as yet vastly in a minority. The masses of mankind are still strongly bound to the flesh pots of Egypt. It is practically impossible to convert these carnivora suddenly from the deeply ingrained meat-eating habit to a strict fruit and vegetable diet. The gradual substitution of vegetable starch and protein for flesh food is easier and safer. A well balanced vegetarian diet, as given in our institution, consisting of combinations of raw relishes, salads, and a moderate amount of cooked foods, is a sufficiently radical change for the majority of those who place themselves under our care and treatment. As they become adapted and accustomed to the vegetarian regimen, we reduce the starches, fats and proteins, and increase the amounts of fruits and vegetables in their dietary until they thoroughly relish the delicate flavours of them.

The Nature Cure Cook Book was planned to serve as a bridge from the customary meat diet to rational vegetarianism and to more radical changes in dietetic habits. It should be in every home in this country, but this desirable consummation cannot be realized if its dietary is too extreme and too restricted along raw food lines. The sooner the convert to vegetarianism learns to reduce starches and proteins to a minimum and to avoid the use of spices and condiments, the better for his health, and the more thoroughly he will learn to enjoy meatless and unfired cookery. The more normal and natural the system, the greater will be the enjoyment of natural food. The gustatory (taste) organs of a body saturated with meat poisons, alcohol, nicotine, caffeine, theobromine, and other food, drink and drug poisons have lost the capacity for sensing and enjoying the delicate flavours of natural food. As the system gradually purifies and the organs of sight, smell and taste become more normal and sensitive, they enjoy more thoroughly the sight, smell and flavour of vegetables, fruits, nuts and cereals — the natural food of man. A diseased body craves abnormal food. The system of drug fiends and alcoholic addicts has to be purified and regenerated by natural foods and treatment before these sufferers can be permanently cured of their unnatural cravings. The transition from the conventional, harmful habits of living in eating, drinking, bathing, exercising and so forth, to the natural ways should not be made too abruptly. It necessitates a gradual re-education of the system from flesh foods to fruits and vegetables, from warm water to cold water bathing, from little or no excercise to systematic, curative gymnastics. Thus we have envisaged throughout the book a graduation from fairly complicated and heavy recipes to simpler ones containing a larger proportion of uncooked food.

CHAPTER 1

WHY WE FAVOUR A VEGETARIAN DIET

We exclude from our dietary the flesh of dead animals because it doubles the work of our organs of elimination and overloads the system with animal waste matter and poisons. The following may serve to explain this more fully:

Two processes are constantly going on in every animal organism — a building up and a tearing down process. The red blood carries into the body the various elements of nutrition and comes back laden with poisonous gases, broken down cell material, and devitalized food products. This debris is carried in the venous blood to the various organs of depuration and excreted in the form of faeces, urine, mucus, perspiration and so forth. Every drop of venous blood and every bit of animal flesh is contaminated with these poisonous excretions of the animal body — the faeces of the cells. The meat eater, therefore, has to eliminate, in addition to his own morbid waste products, those of the animal carcass.

Chemical analysis proves conclusively that uric acid and other uraemic poisons contained in the animal body are almost identical with caffeine, theine and nicotine, the poisonous stimulating properties of coffee, tea and tobacco. This puts flesh foods, meat soups and meat extracts in the same class with tea, coffee, alcohol and tobacco and other poisonous stimulants. It explains why meat stimulates the animal passions and why it creates a craving for liquor, tobacco and other stronger stimulants. Not long ago we saw a father in high glee at the sight of his little two year old baby boy chewing busily at a piece of rare beef steak, the blood running from the corners of his mouth. The father proudly related that the baby already liked his coffee as well as anybody else in the family. Imagine the tender, sensitive nervous system of the little child, from the cradle up, over-irritated with these powerful stimulants. Well informed phsyicians tell us that a very large percentage of children acquire unnatural sexual habits before they leave the public schools. Is it any wonder?

It must also be taken into consideration that the morbid matter of the dead animal body is foreign and uncongenial to the excretory organs of man; in other words, that it is much harder for them to eliminate the waste matter of an animal carcass than that of the human body. Moreover, the formation of ptomaines, or corpse poisons, begins immediately after the death of an animal. This is a serious matter, since meat and poultry are kept in refrigerators for many months and sometimes for years before they reach the kitchen, green and livid looking, and sending forth suspicious odours which have to be doctored with chemicals and spices. The nobler among carnivorous animals devour only freshly slaughtered prey; it remains for scavengers of the hog and hyena type, and for man, to feast on flesh long cold and stark and tainted by the odour of incipient decay.

The foregoing statements will explain why even the best of meats are detrimental to health, but the danger becomes greater when soup, roast, ham or sausage trace their origin to tubercular or "lumpy-jaw" cattle, or to scrofulous or cholera infected hogs. Raw meat is especially dangerous, because it is often the source of trichinae, tapeworms and other parasitic infections. The word scrofula is derived from the Latin word "scrofa" (sow), indicating that the ancients recognized the relationship between eating pork and scrofulous diseases. Even the artificial fattening processes to which the animals are subjected in order to increase their weight and consequent market value are fraught with deleterious effects upon the meat products of their slaughter. It is well recognized that, in most instances, a superabundance of flesh on the human animal is synonymous with systemic poisons and incipient disease. Why should we expect better results from this unnatural and inhuman, though unquestionably "profitable", stuffing treatment inflicted upon cattle, hogs, chickens, and so forth, just prior to their conversion into food for man?

Still other powerful influences tend to poison the flesh of slaughtered animals. It is now well understood that emotions of worry, fear and anger actually poison blood and tissues. Fear and anger of the mother poison her milk and, through the milk, her nursing baby. The bite of an infuriated man has often proved as poisonous as that of a mad dog. All of us have experienced the poisonous and paralyzing effects of worry and fear. Animals are instinctively very sensitive to approaching danger and death. Fear is one of their predominating characteristics. How excited they must be by emotions of worry, anger and fear, after many days of travel, closely packed in shaking cars — hungry, thirsty, tired, scared and angered to the point of madness. Many die before the journey is ended; others are driven, half dead with fear and exhaustion, to the slaughter pens, their instinctive fear of death augmented by the sight and odour of the bloody shambles. Think of the wounded deer and rabbit chased by hounds for many miles before death ends their agonies.

Arguments of the Antis

Arguments in favour of vegetarian diet are usually met with such brilliant objections and criticisms as, "Why did God create cows and hogs if they were not intended for us to eat?" To this thoughtful query we sometimes reply by asking the deeper question, "Why did God create you if you are not to be eaten?" Others tell of the man who eats meat, smokes tobacco, drinks coffee and brandy, and is now four score years old and in perfect health. All are sure that our arguments are mere theories and that nobody can actually prove the truth of our statements.

The fact that some people are so constituted that they can withstand the injurious effects of bad habits for many years does not imply that others can indulge with the same impunity or that hale and hearty ones would not be more hale and hearty without the poisons. Most of these rugged persons owe their iron constitutions to favourable heredity, simple, natural surroundings and frugal fare in early life. Most of them were reared on the farm, or came from the European peasantry who are practically vegetarians. Though these robust ones may endure for a long time the weakening influences of "high living" their offspring have to pay the penalty in bad heredity. Careful observation discloses the interesting fact that the descendants of these hearty pioneers, when exposed to the degenerating influences of our city life become extinct in the third, fourth or fifth generation.([1])

The most direct and positive proof that meat eating is injurious to health and that it prevents the cure of serious chronic ailments comes to us in everyday practice. Some years ago, for instance, there came to see us for treatment a woman whose head was covered on one side by a cancerous mass of large proportions. Her troubles had started two years earlier with an operation for removal of a wen, "because it didn't look well". Neither she nor the learned surgeon, however, took into consideration that behind the wen lurked a constitutional psoric taint, in consequence of which the scar left by the operation soon became inflamed, opened and began to discharge pus. Four different times the wound was operated on, but in spite of antiseptics, cauterization, skin

([1])
It is doubtful whether the robust peasant healthiness to which Lindlahr refers is now found to the same extent in the countries of Western Europe as it was in his day. The use of processed, refined and mass produced foods has spread to the country so that country people grow and produce their own food less than they formerly did. Also it is probable that the quality and food value of much of the produce has declined under modern methods of cultivation.

grafting and everything else the surgeon's skill could do, it would not "stay healed". After the fourth operation the growth became so large and malignant that the surgeons were soon at the end of their wits. They said the growth had developed into a true cancer, and they dismissed the patient as incurable. In this state she came under our treatment and improved rapidly. After five months of natural living and treatment, when scrofula, psora, systemic toxins and drug poisons were thoroughly eliminated from her system, the growth had disappeared and the wound was covered with healthy new skin. Some time after this, however, she returned and reported that the wound had opened once more. On catechizing her we found that — tempted by other members of the family — she had commenced to eat meat. Following our strict advice she again adhered closely to her vegetarian regimen, the wound immediately ceased to discharge and healed once more. Several times after, she had the same experience. Whenever she partook of meat and coffee the wound would open and discharge.

Another case which came under our treatment was that of a man about thirty years of age. When we first attended him in his home he had been in bed with inflammatory rheumatism for five months. He was unable to use his limbs, and his friends had given up all hope of recovery. After four weeks of treatment under our direction at home he was able to come to our sanatorium; two months later he was practically a well man, only there was some inflammation and swelling in his right foot, which made walking very painful. For three months afterward, in spite of vigorous natural treatment, this painful lesion would not yield. Then we became convinced that something was wrong. We told him that somehow he must be violating the law; because if our treatment was good enough to cure the worst of his ailments, this comparatively insignificant symptom should also yield. "Well, doctor," he answered, "I am living strictly to directions, but I have been taking a little meat now and then, and I smoke one or two pipes of tobacco a day. I thought this could not harm me." We explained to him that his system, under the influence of natural living, had become purified to such a degree that it was sensitive now even to small quantities of poison; that there was just enough uric acid and nicotine in the occasional piece of meat and pipe of tobacco to keep the weak part irritated and inflamed. He followed our directions more conscientiously, and from that day the inflammation began to subside. Within a few weeks it disappeared entirely.

Still another phenomenon of common occurrence confirms our opinion that meat eating is neither natural nor necessary to man. People who have eaten meat regularly from childhood adopt and

4

follow under our advice a strictly rational vegetarian diet. After several months of meatless regimen they partake of some tempting roast or fowl and are very much surprised at the result of their experiment. They find that the tempting morsel does not taste as they anticipated. In many instances they experience unpleasant disturbances in their digestive organs, bad taste in the mouth, nausea, diarrhoea, and similar protests against unnatural food. One may cease eating bread, fruits or vegetables for many years, and when these foods are taken again there is never any sign of protest on nature's part; on the contrary, they are relished more than ever.

Persons who have broken and conquered the whiskey or tobacco habit have similar experiences. A glass of whiskey or a cigar taken after a long interval of total abstinence nauseates them as much as when they first began to drink or smoke. They have to learn it all over again. Complaints like the following are quite familiar: "Why, doctor, this simple life is making me so weak that I cannot smoke a cigar without it turning my stomach inside out; it makes me as sick as a green school boy." These acute revulsions are not due to a weakening of the system, but to the fact that the nervous organism is once more sensitive and strong enough to revolt against noxious poisons and forcibly to eliminate them. But, after repeated indulgence, the sensory nerves become so weakened that they can no longer protest, and our backslider is then again "strong enough" to enjoy his steak, smoke, coffee and liquor. In other cases what a glorious experience (for a while) this return to stimulants becomes. The system, under the purifying and relaxing influences of natural living, has become so pure and sensitive that it fully responds to powerful stimulants. Our recreant friend feels so strong and buoyant after a cup of coffee, a smoke or a piece of steak that he "floats on air". He wonders how he could have lived so long without these "wonderful tonics". By and by the scene changes. Brain and nerves becomes paralyzed under the continual action of nicotine, alcohol and uric acid. Morbid matter accumulates and clogs the wheels of life. Bleary eyes, trembling hands, weak heart, rheumatic joints, fagged brain and irritable temper soon tell the result of "eating and drinking what agrees with you". The last state of the backslider is worse than the first. Too often, weakened and discouraged by defeat, he lacks energy and moral courage to make another stand. Physical, mental and moral degeneration are the inevitable results.

"But," I hear somebody ask, "is it not true that meat is the most nutritious of all foods?" This ancient superstition is being rapidly discredited by the investigators of the vitamins. Everywhere scientists of the orthodox school, not at all interested in vegetarianism, are proclaiming that those portions of the animal carcass, commonly used for food, contain only very negligible quantities of vitamins, the mysterious food elements known to be absolutely essential to the maintenance of life and health. Science further claims that the minute and altogether insufficient amounts of these life elements present in flesh foods are destroyed and dissipated by boiling, frying and roasting.

CHAPTER II

IS IT WORTH WHILE TO PAY ATTENTION TO DIET?

Forethought in food selection is indispensible for the restoration and preservation of health, but fear-thought at the table will poison the most wholesome food and drink. As in everything else, it is well to avoid extremes and to stick to the common sense natural way. Many of our modern metaphysicians seem to think that by a sort of mental alchemy they can transmute the elements in their bodies or create them out of nothingness. Divine healers say to us, "Eat and drink what you please; pray; the Lord will make it all right". The Christian Scientist says, "Diatetics is a snare and a delusion. Foods cannot harm you as long as you do not think they can." I doubt whether the Lord has the time or the inclination continually to make good the bad results of wrong eating, over-feeding, and food poisoning. Neither is the advice of the doctor and the Christian Scientist, "Eat what agrees with you", in keeping with the dictates of common sense, or with the findings of science. No matter what we try to produce, whether it be an apple pie, a picture, a locomotive or a phonograph, we know that in the making of these or any other things we require certain materials in certain well defined proportions. But how many people apply this self evident principle to the management of their bodies?

The wonderfully constructed human machine is also composed of certain materials in well defined proportions, of which, so far, seventeen have been discovered by chemical science. If any of these are present in overabundance, and others are deficient or wholly lacking, there will surely result abnormal structure and function, in other words, disease. The normal composition of vital fluids and tissues depends upon the food and drink which is taken into the system. Therefore, the elements of nutrition must be provided in right proportions in order to supply the needs of the body. But is it not a fact that most people pay no attention whatever to these obvious truths? They take into their long-suffering stomachs any odd combinations of food materials without the slightest consideration as to whether they will meet the manifold requirements of the human organism. The only question in the selection of food seems to be, "Does it taste good?". Then people wonder why they are afflicted with dyspepsia, chronic constipation, appendicitis, cancer and the multitude of other ailments resulting from malnutrition and autointoxication. The majority of medical practitioners do not seem to know any more about the principles of natural dietetics than the laity. Their advice on diet runs about as follows: "Do not pay any attention to food faddists — there is no exact science of dietetics — what is one man's food is another man's poison — eat what agrees with you — take plenty of good nourishing food — the only safe guide to food selection is appetite and instinct", and so on. Such is the wisdom dispensed by certain popular writers on hygiene and dietetics, who, blessed with more conceit than scientific knowledge, ridicule the idea and deny the possibility of an exact science of dietetics.

"Eat what agrees with you." If this be good and true advice, then caffeine must be good for the coffee toper, nicotine for the smoker, alcohol for the drunkard, and morphine, cocaine and opium, for the dope fiend. For these poisons seem to "agree" exceedingly well with the people habitually addicted to their use. If suddenly deprived of their favourite stimulants or narcotics, they suffer great distress, become very ill, and may even die as the result of such deprivation. These are the people who say, "I never eat fruits and vegetables. They taste flat; they do not agree with me; they actually sicken me." This would seem to indicate that for the majority of human beings, taste, appetite and cravings are not safe guides. The following explains why this is so. The animal, living in freedom, is guided in the selection of its food as well as in all other of its life habits by instinct, that is, by the wisdom of Mother Nature. Therefore, the animal acts in accordance with the laws of its being and, as a result of this, possesses perfect health, strength and beauty, preserves its faculties, capacities and powers almost to the very end of its life and then dies an easy, painless, natural death. Guided by nature, the animal selects and partakes of only those foods which are best suited to its particular constitution. The lion does not eat grass, nor the cow devour the bleeding carcass of a lamb. Each animal adheres to a limited combination of foods best adapted to its individual needs. The only exception to this are a few omnivorous scavengers, such as the hyena, vulture, hog and chicken;

7

for them nothing seems too vile to swallow. The nobler carnivorous animals, as the lion, tiger, leopard, and so forth, live only on freshly killed meat. They would not touch the carcass of a dead and decaying animal. The gourmand prefers his game when it is tainted with putrefaction. In the course of evolutionary development, man has lost the animal instinct and therewith the faculty for natural food selection. Reason, which took the place of instinct, was, in the past, not enlightened enough to be a trustworthy guide in regulating life habits. Instead of living in harmony with nature's laws, man catered to his perverted appetites. In order to produce artificial stimulation, he learned to use spices and condiments, to convert wholesome grains and delicious grapes into alcohol. He became addicted to the use of the poisonous xanthines and alkaloids of tea, coffee, tobacco and narcotic drugs. Such artificial stimulation of the taste buds in the tongue and of the sensory nerves inevitably results in gradual atrophy and loss of their natural sensitiveness, and this calls for still stronger stimulants to "tickle" the paralysed nerves and the no longer sensitive palate. It is for these reasons that people addicted to the use of spices, condiments, stimulants and narcotics have lost the capacity for sensing and enjoying the most delicate aromas and flavours of fruits and vegetables.

This brings us to the question: "What is Natural Food?". We have endeavoured to define this term as follows: Natural food for animals and man is that food which appeals to the senses of sight, taste and smell in the natural condition, as it comes from nature's hands. Any food which needs disguising by cooking, spicing and pickling is not "natural". For instance, fruits, berries, nuts, vegetables and grains can be eaten with relish in the uncooked state by healthy normal individuals. This is true even of raw potatoes, carrots, beets and other roots which are enjoyed and perfectly digested by healthy children. On the other hand, raw meat, uncooked and unspiced, is revolting to the sensory organs. Before it can be relished, the taste and smell of the corpse must be disguised by boiling, roasting and much seasoning. People who have been heavy meat eaters all their lives, after living on a vegetarian diet for a few months frequently acquire a strong dislike for the odour of raw meat and even for the odour and taste of cooked meat. This is not true in the case of grains, roots, fruits and vegetables. The longer a person is forced to abstain from them, the more they are needed and relished.

In making the foregoing statements, it is not our intention to force our readers to strict vegetarianism. But as we proceed in our discussions we shall endeavour to point out the advantages and disadvantages of different foods and food combinations. The reader can then form his own conclusions and put the theories here presented to the test of practical experience. Someone might say: "The study of food chemistry and scientific dietetics is too difficult for the ordinary individual. We have to leave these things to the doctors." This is a mistake. Natural Therapeutics has reduced the art and science of natural dietetics to such simplicity that they can be comprehended and applied by anyone endowed with ordinary intelligence. The quest after a normal, natural diet is not as silly and impossible as some people would make you believe.

Starving America is the title of a very instructive book on food chemistry and food poisoning, by Alfred W. McCann. This publication shows how rapidly the teachings of Nature Cure are spreading in this country, for all the author's important arguments and statements dealing with food chemistry were fully treated in our articles in the *Nature Cure Magazine* in the period from 1907 to 1909. The expression "Starving America" indeed sounds rather strange. Is it possible that this glorious country of ours, blessed more abundantly by Mother Nature than any other, the richest on God's footstool, can be starving amidst a plethora of all that human beings need to live and thrive on in comfort and luxury (provided its products were justly distributed)? Yes, it is not only possible, but an actual fact that America is starving amidst plenty; not only its inhabitants are starving, but in many localities the soil as well. What is strangest of all, those who have the greatest abundance in lands and money are starving just as surely as are the underpaid and overworked wage earners. In many ways the wealthy are worse off than the poor, because they are not only starved, but also poisoned by overabundance of food and of leisure. You ask: "What is the meaning of all this nonsense?" It is this: The people of America have been overfed with starches, sugars, fats and nitrogenous foods (meat, eggs and glutens), but starved from lack of the all important mineral elements – the organic salts and vitamins — on which depend absolutely the normal structure and functions of the body, or physical and mental health. The public in general, as well as the medical schools, have been ignorant on the subject of true food values and of true food chemistry. Doctors and laymen have laboured under the mistaken idea that the only food worth considering because of their nutritional value, are the starches, sugars, fats and proteins. The most recent works on dietetics, used in our best medical schools, take into consideration these foods only. They have nothing to say on the importance of the mineral elements in the economy of the human body and science is only just awakening to the existence and importance of the vitamins or life elements. As yet it has not become

9

generally known that certain alkaline mineral elements, though present only in minute quantities in foods and in animal and human bodies are essential to life and health. If these tissue salts are lacking in the food, and if, as a result of this, they are deficient in the body, disease is bound to arise; and in this event, overfeeding on the nourishing starches, sugars, fats and proteins will serve only to make matters worse. These statements are, of course, contrary to popular notions and to the pseudoscientific teachings of the schools. They say, "If a person be weak, sickly and emaciated, stuff him with plenty of rich, nourishing food." This is held to be good and common sense practice; but what is the usual result? The "stuffed" anaemic grows weaker and thinner, and the "stuffing" of the consumptive serves only to make his condition more hopeless. The very abundance of meat and eggs, which is supposed to build up these patients, poisons their systems beyond the possibility of recovery.

To be sure, starches, sugars, fats and proteins meet certain demands and fill very important functions in the economy of the body, but, on the other hand, they produce in the processes of digestion large amounts of poisonous acids, alkaloids, gases and ptomaines. To these morbid by-products of digestion are added the excretions or faeces of the cells. Furthermore, the cells and tissues of the body are constantly changing, building up and breaking down, just like the body as a whole. The broken down tissue materials also create large quantities of morbid matter and poisons. Practically all disease arising in the human organism is caused originally by the accumulation of these effete waste and end-products of digestion and of the tissue changes. Therefore, in order to ensure normal structure and functions, in other words, good health, these waste products must be neutralized and eliminated from the system as promptly and completely as possible. This neutralization and elimination depends upon an abundant supply in blood and tissues of the alkaline mineral elements, also called nutritious salts or tissue salts, the most important of which are iron, sodium, lime, lithium, magnesium, manganese, potassium and silicon. These mineral elements are found in all the important secretions of the body. Upon them depends the richness of the blood and the solidity of the fleshy and bony structures. They are the building stones of the physical organism.

The science of biochemistry deals with the functions of these mineral salts in the life activities of the ascending kingdoms of nature; the mineral, the vegetable, the animal and the human. Upon this science is based rational soil feeding as well as the biochemic treatment of diseases by means of tissue salts, vito-chemical, homoeopathic and herbal remedies. Natural diet or rational vegetarianism is based, also, upon this strictly scientific foundation. The medicinal values of the natural foods and remedies depend upon their richness in the positive mineral elements and vitamins.

The foregoing explains why our American people are starving in the midst of plenty. Their "highly nutritious" and "luxurious" meat-potato-white bread-coffee-and-pie diet contains an overabundance of the poison-producing, negative food elements of the first four groups, but it is altogether deficient in the positive, alkaline, mineral elements of the fifth group, which are the carriers of the Vitamins. (see Dietetics in a Nutshell, page 35).

CHAPTER III

FOR WHAT DO WE EAT AND DRINK?

The majority of people would reply: "Why everybody knows that from food and drink we derive our strength." Are you sure of this? Do you really believe that the large amount of animal heat and vital energy which the human body manufactures, radiates and expends every twenty-four hours is derived from a few pounds of food consumed in the course of a day? Any hard working labourer or athlete spends an enormous amount of power and energy every day. A healthy individual may continue to do this for several weeks without taking any food whatever. The best proof that not all the heat and muscular energy of the body are derived from the combustion of food materials is furnished by the long fast. Of late years, since fasting has become popular as a natural remedy, many thousands of people have fasted from four to ten weeks at a stretch. The majority of these Marathon fasters report but slight loss in physical energy. Many claim that they are stronger at the end of the fast than at the beginning. The loss in animal heat is negligible. While in some instances the temperature declines a fraction of a degree, or a degree, in the majority of cases it remains normal. We have verified this in hundreds of cases under close observation, in our institutions. To cite cases from personal observation: One of our patients suffering from typhoid malaria did not take any food except water for seven weeks. At the end of that time his body temperature was normal. During the last two weeks of the fast he lost only two pounds. Another patient afflicted with cancer of the stomach lived for two years on a few ounces of food daily, mostly white of egg and fruit juices. His temperature was normal almost to the last.

Whether sweltering under the tropical sun of the equator or freezing with arctic cold, the temperature of the body is exactly the same. If it drops or rises a few degrees below or above normal, death ensues. This regulation of the bodily heat, regardless of the surrounding temperature, and, within certain limits, regardless of the quantity and quality of food consumed is one of the greatest mysteries of the wonderful human organism. If foods were the only source of animal heat and working energy, fasting for a long period would be impossible; the temperature would sink below normal soon after the commencement of the fast. It may be said that while abstaining from food the body lives on itself — that it consumes its own tissues; this, however, does not account for the production of all the heat and energy expended during a long fast. In a number of cases under our observation, the average loss of weight during a forty-nine day fast did not amount to more than thirty-two pounds — approximately two-thirds of a pound a day. This is not sufficient fuel material to provide for the enormous radiation of heat and the expenditure of muscular energy of the human body during twenty-four hours.

Is Food the True and Only Source of Vital Energy?

In order to understand this all important problem more fully let us study for a moment what combustion is. The process of burning, combustion, fermentation, digestion, rusting, decaying and putrefaction, are similar in nature. They are all processes of oxidation. They differ only in rapidity of action. They all represent the breaking down of complex materials into simpler forms through the combination of the oxygen in the air with the carbon in the oxidizing materials. This disintegration is accompanied by the chemical combination of the oxygen of the air with the carbon, the iron, or some other element of the burning, fermenting, putrefying, or rusting substance. During these processes of disintegration, the carbon recombines with the oxygen of the air (combustion) and the latent life energy and sun heat are liberated, furnishing heat, light and other forms of energy.

The Sources of Animal Heat

A man may eat in the right proportions all the seventeen chemical elements found in his body. He may also take a sufficient amount of air and water. Yet, if taken in pure mineral form, he will die almost immediately because some of these elements, instead of nourishing him, will act on him as powerful poisons. Experiments carried on by many food scientists have demonstrated that even proximate food elements, such as starch, fat and protein, when chemically pure, will not sustain animal or human life. Animals fed on chemically pure starch or white sugar die sooner than those which receive no food at all. This clearly indicates that the various chemical elements found in food and drink, do not in and by themselves sustain animal and human life, but that life, heat and energy depend on something more than these.

What is this mysterious something which builds up and sustains vegetable, animal and human bodies? The majority of scientists assume that the sun supplies all heat and energy on our planet; that sun light and sun heat are the only sources of vegetable and animal energy. The fallacy of their reasoning is due to the fact that the forces and energies latent in and proceeding from the sun are not by any means the highest expression of life or vital force on this planet. That which we call "life", which animates the entire created universe, is the primary source of all forces and all energies. Sun energy is merely a manifestation of this primary force of all forces, which manifests with increasing potency in the ascending kingdoms of nature. This primary life force or vital force manifests in the mineral kingdom as the electro-magnetic life element, in the vegetable kingdom as the vito-chemical life element, in the animal kingdom as the spiritual life element, and in the human kingdom as the soul life element. These life elements, in conjunction with the light and heat (radio active forces) of the sun, elaborate the elements of the earth and air into the ascending forms of the four kingdoms of nature. In other words, life or vital force is the builder, while sun energy is only one of the building materials; life force is primary, sun energy is secondary. The more powerful the vital energy which builds, the more potent are the latent dynamics or potential force of the products. Coal, though classed among the minerals, possesses greater heat and energy producing qualities than other minerals, because originally its molecules were elaborated under the influence of the vito-chemical or vegetable life element. The animal cell, being built up under the operation of the spiritual or animal life element, is alive with still higher potencies of vital force than those latent in the vegetable cell.

The energy which builds up molecules becomes bound or latent in that which it builds. This is illustrated in the formation of ice and coal. The low temperature which solidifies the molecules of water is absorbed and becomes bound or latent in the icy crystals which it builds. When the particles of ice disintegrate under the influence of warmer temperature, "cold" is liberated in our refrigerator. In similar

13

manner, the heat which gives warmth and comfort to our homes in the winter time is vital force (vito-chemical), plus the sunlight and sun heat which were absorbed in the formation of vegetable cells in the growing plants and trees of primaeval forests. Vital force corresponds to fire; food corresponds to fuel. If the life force has departed from an animal or human body, no amount of food can create animal heat. As the fuel in the furnace has to be consumed by fire before it can liberate heat, so the food in the body has to be consumed by the life force before its latent heat and energy can be liberated. When in the processes of digestion and assimilation the latent energies stored in the food have been liberated and absorbed by the body nothing remains of the erstwhile food but poisonous excrements which, if not properly eliminated, become destructive to the organism — the organic has become inorganic. When the life principle is taken away from food materials nothing remains but waste and poison. Vegetable and animal food are therefore foods only by virtue of the vital and solar energy locked up in their molecules. As soon as the vegetables or animal molecules disintegrate by any process whatsoever, their vital energy is dissipated and lost. This explains why cooking wastes food energy; why fermentation changes wholesome foods into poisonous alcohol; why "predigested foods" are weakened foods. The meddling arts of the cook, chemist and distiller, therefore, seldom improve nature's foods, and the chemist's dream, that all foods will some day be made in his laboratory and handed out in tablet form, will always remain a dream.

Among the modern writers who boldly defend the mechanical theory of vital force, no-one has done more ingenious work than Dr. Thomas Powell in his interesting book, *Fundamentals and Requirements of Health and Disease.* We shall quote and discuss his theory in order to contrast the mechanical and vital conceptions of vital force and also to give his ingenious theory of the production of muscular energy. Among other startling claims, he asserts that he has discovered the nature and *modus operandi* of vital, or, as he calls it, "vito-motive" force. The substance of his theory is this: The red, arterial blood stores carbonaceous compounds in the interior of the hollow muscle fibrils. When the ego wills to move a muscle, the mind (will) sends a nerve spark to the muscle fibrils. This ignites, or explodes, the C O H molecules stored in the fibrils. The combustion of the carbon compounds produces carbonic acid. The carbonic acid expands the muscle fibril into a round, balloon-like shape. This shortens or contracts the fibrils lengthwise. The contraction of the muscle fibrils also contracts the muscle fascia, and the muscle in its entirety. Therefore, he claims that carbonic acid is the mysterious vito-motive power which so long has eluded the search of scientists.

In order to present his theory correctly, we shall quote a few paragraphs from his book.

"The facts which are involved in the transformation of the potential energy of the food into the kinetic form, as we find it in the vito-motive power, cannot be too deeply impressed upon the mind; hence it will be well to repeat: 1. The nutrient matter stored in the cells in the consummation of the nutritive process, consisting as it does of a most intimate comminglement of food and oxygen — of a combustible with a supporter of combustion — is in a state of extremely unstable equilibrium, and is, therefore, nothing more nor less than a delicately balanced explosive of high potential; 2. The carbon and oxygen thus intimately associated is brought into chemical combination by act of the will expressed by means of the nerves and nervous influence; 3. Whenever the will so orders, an explosion must occur in every cell which is included in or reached by the volitional edict; 4. The carbon dioxide thus generated within the cells forces them to expand and in a direction which is transverse to the long axis of the fibril, this being the line of least resistance, as above explained; 5. The expanding cells impinge upon the inner surface of the fascia, forcing it to yield in like manner and for the same reason, thus producing that transverse expansion and longitudinal shortening of the muscle on which the activities of the body chiefly and evidently depend, as above stated. In short, the will acts, the nutrient matter explodes, the cells expand, the fascia yields, the muscle contracts, and the vital machinery is set in motion; not, however, in consequence of "metabolism" of the "white blood corpuscle", but of the red; not by reason of the "metamorphosis" of the tissues of the body, but of food; not by the energy of "resurrected sunbeams" nor of any other immaterial agency, but of expanding carbon dioxide gas; not in consequence of the presence of nitrogen in the food nor of any other incombustible element, but of carbon, and this is not from the inorganic world, but the organic; not by a product of any laboratory of human origin, but of the plant world — that immeasurably greater concern which was instituted by the All Wise Being, and for the express purpose of effecting the separation of those elements — carbon and oxygen — from whose reunion within the nutritive cells of the living organism must come all the energies, physical, nervous and thermal, of the entire domain of animated nature.

"It shows that the doctrine of *vis vitae*, held by Liebig and his contemporaries, and recently revised to some extent, is utterly erroneous; that while it is true that there is an ego or inherent vital principle, it is also true that the movements of the living organism are due to the intra-cellular production and action of the vito-motive power — that energy displaying agent which is known to science as carbon dioxide or carbonic acid gas."

We do not understand why Dr. Powell does not give hydrogen as well as the carbonic acid credit for the work performed in the muscle fibrils. In the combustion of carbonaceous compounds, such as glycogen, dextrose, glucose and haemoglobin, a great deal of hydrogen is liberated, as well as carbonic acid, and the former gas is more powerful to expand balloons than is carbonic acid. If Dr. Powell's ingenious theory of muscle inflation and contraction by carbonic acid is true he has discovered the *modus operandi* of carbon combustion in so far as it is concerned in the production of muscular energy. But he has failed to discover the great life force which elaborates the carbon compounds in the vegetable and animal kingdoms and which ignites and explodes them in the cells and muscle fibrils of animal and human bodies. If no immaterial agency is concerned in the production of muscular labour and of animal heat, how does he explain that these manifestations of kinetic energy suddenly cease when the life element departs, when death takes place? When the body is dead muscle labour and heat production cease, though the corpse be heated far beyond the normal temperature of the living body, and though the material elements for the production of heat and energy are present as before. The question which the doctor has failed to answer is: What is it that makes possible the combustion of the carbon compounds and the production of carbonic gas? Elated over the discovery of the very last stage of muscle labour, he ignores the Intelligence and Power which created the fuel material as well as the wonderful organism which consumes it — the *Life* or *Vital Force* which animates the atom as well as solar systems and their sentient inhabitants.

It is not true that carbonic acid is the great vito-motive force. The gas may be the motive force in the rendering of muscle labour, but the nerve spark which produces it through igniting the carbon compounds, and the mind and will which release the nerve spark or impulse are much nearer and more potent expressions of the great *Life Force* than is carbonic acid gas. After all, our conception of the nature of vito-motive force as summed up in the following sentence is more rational: All forms of energy which manifest in the mineral, vegetable, animal and human entities are secondary energies, derived from the primary source of all forces, powers and energies in the sidereal universe, from that which we call God, Life, Oversoul, Universal Intelligence, Great Spirit, Buddha, Prana and so forth, each according to his own highest conception and best understanding. This is the *vis vitae*, the *animus*

16

mundi, ignored and denied by the speculative sophistries of materialistic science, but recognized and described by Swedenborg as the Heat of Divine Love and the Light of Divine Wisdom, radiating from the Great Central Sun of the Universe through all space and animating all things.

The True Source of Vital Energy

The question will be asked: "If we do not derive our vital energy from food and drink, why is it that we die when we cease eating and drinking?" The answer to this has already been given. The only rational explanation is that vegetable, animal and human bodies are contrivances for the transmutation of life force into the various working energies or life elements which manifest in the ascending kingdoms of nature. To illustrate: A windmill is a contrivance for transforming the potential energy of the moving winds into kinetic or working energy which drives the machinery of the mill. The resistance offered by the sails of a ship transmutes the potential energy of the air currents into kinetic energy which propels the vessel. The earth is a contrivance for converting the radio active emanations of the sun into warmth and light which makes possible the existence of life on our planet. The sun sends forth these radio active emanations into open space in all directions, but unless intercepted and obstructed by a solid planetary body they do not transform the darkness and coldness of interplanetary space into heat and light. In similar manner, mineral, vegetable, animal and human bodies are contrivances for the transmutation of omnipresent life force into the various energies of life elements which animate all things in the ascending kingdoms of nature. If they do not give life, what, then, are the functions of food and drink in the economy of the body? All they can do is to furnish the materials to keep the system in such a condition that vital force can manifest in and through it. The inflow of the life force into the cells and organs of the body and its free distribution by way of the nervous system, depends upon a normal healthy condition of the organism. Anything and everything in natural methods of living and treatment that will help to build up the blood on a normal basis, that will purify the system of waste and morbid matter, that will correct mechanical lesions and harmonize mental and emotional conditions, will insure a greater supply of life force and its derivatives, strength, vitality, resistance and recuperative power. In other words, the more normal, healthy and perfect the organism, the more copious will be the inflow of vital energy.

Never before in any writings dealing with dietetics or food chemistry has there been revealed the true relationship between the life force and food, medicines, tonics and stimulants.

CHAPTER IV

THE NORMAL FUNCTIONS OF FOOD AND DRINK IN THE ECONOMY OF THE BODY

Foods build and foods destroy. First we shall study the normal beneficial effects of food, then the harmful and destructive. Food and drink perform the following functions in the vital processes of the body:

(1) They furnish the amount of water necessary to hold in solution the constituent elements of the body and to make possible the circulation of the vital fluids and the elimination of waste and morbid matter.

(2) They supply bulk, in the form of cellulose and woody fibre, which offers solid resistance to the intestines, thereby stimulating the peristaltic movements of the bowels and acting as scourers, purifiers and laxatives.

(3) They provide fuel materials.

(4) They provide materials for the building and repair of the tissues of the body in the form of proteins and amino-acids.

(5) They supply the positive mineral salts, which are important as building materials, as neutralizers and eliminators of poisonous acids, alkaloids and ptomaines, and as producers and conductors of the electromagnetic energies in the system.

(6) They supply vitamins or life elements.

We shall now consider separately the various functions of food materials in the economy of the body in connection with our classification of foods.

GROUP I.   Starches (COH)
GROUP II.   Dextrins and Sugars (COH)

The foods belonging to these two groups are called carbohydrates, because their essential elements are carbon and hydrogen. When chemically pure they are composed of carbon, hydrogen and oxygen. The oxygen and hyrdogen occur in proportions which form water (H_2O). These foods are to the human body what the fuel is to a furnace; they are producers of heat and energy. Through the processes of digestion the starches are changed into dextrins and glucose, cane sugar into levulose, the milk sugar into galactose, which are absorbed in the digestive tract. Starches can enter the circulation of the blood, through the cell linings of the intestines, only in the form of levulose and galactose. Unless the starches are transformed into these highly refined sugars they remain not only useless for purposes of nutrition, but their partially fermented debris gives rise to mucoid clogging and obstruction of the intestinal membranes, and to putrefactive fermentation, gas formation, and systemic poisoning. These highly refined sugars are burned up in the muscular tissues, and produce heat and muscular energy in a manner not understood by orthodox science. Dr. Thomas Powell's interesting explanation of the *modus operandi* of glucose in the production of muscular energy has been given in the last chapter.

Glycogen, or Animal Starch

If more sugars are consumed and absorbed than the system can immediately use for the production of heat and muscular energy, the surplus is changed in the liver into glycogen. This "animal starch", as it has been called, is stored in the liver until needed for the production of heat and muscular energy, and then released in the form of glucose. Therefore, it appears that the liver is a storehouse for the fuel materials of the body. The expenditure of glucose by the liver is regulated by certain secretions from the pancreas. The pancreas thus acts as a regulator, or brake, on the sugar production of the liver. If the sugar inhibiting influence of the pancreas is interfered with by disease of this organ, diabetes follows. This has been proved conclusively by experiments on animals. If the pancreas is removed, the blood stream immediately becomes saturated with sugar, and death takes place within a few days from diabetic coma.

Practically all writers on food chemistry, including vegetarians, claim that sun heat and energy, latent in carbonaceous foods, is the only source of heat and energy in animal and human bodies. This, however, as we have pointed out in another chapter, is a great mistake which has led to many false conclusions and harmful practices — especially to overeating and the taking of poisonous stimulants and tonics under the mistaken idea that vital energy can be increased in that way. The fallacy of this conception of the source of animal heat and energy we have explained in the previous chapter.

GROUP III.   (F) Fats and Oils (COH)

To this group of food materials belong all oils and fats. They are called hydrocarbons, because they, also, are chemically composed of carbon, hydrogen and oxygen — but the hydrogen and oxygen are not in proportions which form water (H_2O). The melting of sugar liberates water, the melting of fats does not — it produces oil only.

In the vital processes of the body, fats and oils also serve as producers of heat and energy. Aside from this they act as lubricants for the digestive tract. Another "new discovery" of Dr. Powell is that fats are not proper food; that fats, as such, have no food value for the human body.

19

This theory, however, seems fallacious, because nature, in milk and eggs, provides fats for the new-born animal and human and for the un-hatched chick, in considerable quantities. We would rather trust the wisdom of nature in such matters than the far-fetched theories and "new discoveries" of writers on food chemistry. It has moreover been found that the fats of milk and eggs are exceedingly rich in fat soluble A vitamin.

GROUP IV.   (P) Proteins or Nitrogenous Foods (COHNPS)

The principle representatives of this group are the lactalbumin of milk, albumen (white of egg), myosin (the flesh of animals), gluten (the dark outer part of cereals), the globulin of the blood and many other forms of protein food materials found in plants, and animal bodies. The simplest forms of protein matter are made up of carbon, oxygen, hydrogen and nitrogen. The more complex forms in addition to these four basic elements, contain phosphorus and sulphur. From the chemical composition of proteins it will be seen that, like the food materials of the first, second and third groups, they contain the COH molecule and can, therefore, take the place of starches, dextrins and sugars, as producers of heat and energy. But in addition to these func-tions, proteins serve other very important purposes in the metabolism (vital economy) of the body. Vegetable, animal and human cells are composed of protoplasm, which means protein matter. The building and repair of these cells, therefore, depends on a sufficient supply of protein food materials. It is for this reason that starches, sugars and fats cannot entirely take the place of nitrogenous foods.

Amino-Acids

Protein food elements are highly complex substances and vary greatly in their qualities of nutrition. It was found that some promote growth and flesh formation in growing animals and humans; others do not. When this was discovered further research revealed that protein food elements are made up of many chemical units, called amino-acids, in much the same way as words are made up of letters. Just as the twenty-six letters of the alphabet can be used to construct many differ-ent words, so the seventeen or more amino-acids obtained by the chemical subdivision of proteins make up various forms of protein food elements, such as the gluten of cereals, casein of milk, albumen of the egg, haemoglobin of the red blood corpuscle, and so forth. Some of the most important of these amino-acids for growth and the mainten-ance of health and weight are the tyrosin and tryptophane in milk and eggs and the lysin, edestin, globulin and glutenin in fruits and vegetables.

20

When mysosin, the protein constituent of meat, is acted upon by the digestive juices of the stomach and intestines, it is broken up into its component amino-acids. This digestion, or decomposition, is necessary before absorption and assimilation can take place. Protein directly introduced into the blood acts like a poison; but after the enzymes, or digestive ferments in the stomach and intestines, have reduced the complex protein material into amino-acids, then these chemical units or building stones are rebuilt into protein substances needed for cell repair and cell growth. This rebuilding of amino-acids into protein materials takes place in the cell linings of the intestinal tract and in the internal cells, tissues and organs of the body. The question may be asked: "Why is it necessary that proteins should be broken down into their units if they are rebuilt at once into new protein substances?" This is necessary in order to enable the cells and cell colonies in the tissues and organs of the body to select and combine such protein substances as they need for building and repair materials. The same letters will make many different words, and many different buildings can be made of the same kind of bricks, all according to the way in which they are combined. Proteins vary greatly as to the number and qualities of the amino-acids which they contain, thus supplying the various needs of animal and human bodies. The question may be asked: "Would it not simplify matters if nature furnished the eighteen or more amino-acids necesary for cell life and growth in simple units instead of highly complex combinations?". Nature may do this for the same reason that many different foods are sold in one store. Each cell selects that which it needs, and rejects the rest. These discoveries verified by many experiments, reveal the fact that quality of protein is just as important and in many respects more important than quantity.

During the period of general food shortage following the Napoleonic war, French scientists extracted gelatin from the bones of animal carcasses, believing that this cheap protein product would take the place of the more expensive meat and cereal protein foods. It was found, however, that the gelatin thus produced not only failed to maintain health but that, if entirely depended upon to take the place of ordinary protein food, it soon brought about weakness, sickness, and death. This may be accounted for, however, by the fact that in the process of manufacture the protein of the bones was robbed of its mineral elements and vitamins, in a similar way to that which takes place in the manufacture of white sugar, polished rice and white flour. Of late years further experiments with gelatin and other non-vitamin food substances revealed just what forms of amino-acids are essential to sustain animals in normal condition, and to promote growth and flesh produc-

21

tion. While gelatin, plus carbohydrates (sugar), plus mineral salts (extracted from milk), were found to be insufficient to sustain animals in health and flesh, an addition to this diet of two amino-acids, tyrosin and tryptophane, met all requirements, and kept the animals in good condition. In similar manner it was found that the amino-acids lysin and edestin, are necessary, in addition to tyrosin and tryptophane, in order to promote growth and normal development of flesh in new-born and growing animals and babies.

We now come to the most important conclusions derived from these researches. The following forms of protein are essential to promote growth in rats: Casein and lactalbumin in milk, ovalbumin and ovovitellin in eggs, excelsin of nuts, edestin and globulin of vegetables and of cotton seed, glutelin of wheat and maize, and glycinin of soy-bean. Proteins which may contribute to maintenance of normal conditions but which fail to induce growth are: the leguminin and legumin of beans and peas, gleadin of wheat and rye, hordein of barley, zein of maize, and phaselin of white kidney beans. The protein of lean meat is not mentioned by scientific experimenters as conducive to growth. However, it probably contains small amounts of the animal proteins contained in milk and in eggs. Very interesting in this respect is the fact that the muscular parts of the animal carcass usually used for food do not contain sufficient amino-acids and vitamins to sustain health and life. This is fully demonstrated and explained in the chapters dealing with the "Nature and Source of Vitamins". In this connection it is very significant that the same foods which carry the growth-promoting amino-acids also contain the vitamins essential to growth and normal development. This seems to indicate that the growth-promoting amino-acids enumerated above carry the growth-promoting vitamins. From the foregoing it becomes apparent that it is good policy not to depend in our vegetarian or natural diet on one or a few forms of protein; that it is best to use a variety of those proteins which are most favourable to the promotion of growth, production of flesh and maintenance of health and strength.

These revelations of scientific research again verify and confirm many of the teachings of Natural Therapeutics. We have always advocated and urged the liberal use of the dairy products, eggs and honey, on account of the "animal magnetism" which they contain. On the other hand, we have always warned against the excessive use of legumes, "because they contain too much protein and not enough of the mineral salts and life elements". We have no doubt that the proteins of legumes and cereals classified as non-growth-producing are identical with those constituents that are robbed of mineral matter and vitamins in the modern milling and refining processes. These revelations also justify our opposition to a strict, raw food diet, mono-diet, or any other extreme dietetic regimen. We always maintained that a moderate variety in food selection and combination was advisable in order to give the cells and tissues a better chance for appropriate food selection.

GROUP V.   (M) Positive Mineral Elements

To this group belong all food materials which run low in acid forming carbohydrates, hydrocarbons and proteins of the first four groups, but high in the positive alkaline mineral elements, the most important of which are iron, sodium, lime, potassium, magnesium and manganese. The old school of medicine considers fruits and vegetables of no importance because they do not contain enough of the "highly nutritious" starches, fats and proteins. We now understand why, just because of this and by virtue of their high percentages of acid binding, positive mineral elements, the fruits and vegetables are of the greatest importance in the economy of the body. Besides being the neutralizers and eliminators of morbid materials, the positive elements are the principal components of the blood and of the most important secretions of the body. One half of the substance of the body structure consists of lime. Potassium is to the muscular tissues what lime is to the bones. These mineral elements are the building stones in the tissues of the body, while the protein elements are the mortar. A wall built with mortar alone cannot stand; it will soon crumble to pieces. The stones embedded in the mortar are necesary to give it tensile strength. So the strength, resistance and stamina of the tissues of the body depend upon the mineral and earthy elements. Deficiency of these causes anaemia, rachitis, scurvy, haemophilia, beriberi, pellagra, decay of teeth and pyorrhoea.

Polarity

Furthermore, the generation of positive electricity and magnetism in the body depends upon an abundance of the positive mineral elements in the circulation. Health is positive; disease negative. When the negative elements are in preponderance, weakness and disease, both physical and mental are bound to result. From the foregoing it becomes apparent why in our natural diet we endeavour to reduce the negative food materials of the first four groups and to increase the positive alkaline mineral elements of the fifth group.

Bulk

There is still another reason why fruits and vegetables, together with the hulls of grains, are of great importance in the processes of digestion and elimination. These food materials contain large amounts of cellulose and woody fibre, which are looked upon ordinarily as useless waste, but in reality render valuable services. They stimulate in a natural manner the peristaltic movements of the bowels and act as scourers and purifiers and, therefore, as natural laxatives.

Vitamins or Life Elements

These essential food elements, their true source, characteristic and functions in the vital economy are fully described in later chapters.

CHAPTER V

THE DESTRUCTIVE EFFECTS OF FOOD AND DRINK

If foods had no other effects than those so far described in this chapter there would be no problem of dietetics. We could do like the majority of people — eat and drink what tastes good — and not bother our heads about scientific food combinations. Any ordinary food mixture would satisfy the needs of the body. But we find that, aside from their beneficial effects upon the organism, these foods, in the processes of digestion, liberate certain waste and morbid materials, which, if allowed to accumulate in considerable quantities in the tissues of the body, endanger health and life. These morbid by-products and end-products of starchy, fatty and protein digestion consist largely of poisonous acids, alkaloids and ptomaines. This is explained by the fact that all the six elements (COHNPS) which make up the food materials in the first four groups are electromagnetically negative, acid-forming elements. In the processes of digestion and oxidation, the foods are torn apart and divided into their component and proximate elements that enter into new combinations, many of which, when they accumulate in the human body, become obstructive and destructive. To elucidate this more fully, we shall quote a few paragraphs from the *Philosophy of Natural Therapeutics*.

"Nearly every disease originating in the human body is due to or accompanied by the excessive formation of different kinds of acids or other pathogenic substances in the system. These are formed during the processes of protein and starch digestion and in the waste products of cells and tissues. Of these various waste products uric acid probably causes the most trouble in the organism. The majority of diseases arising within the human body are due to its erratic behaviour. Together with oxalic acid and oxylates it is responsible for arteriosclerosis, rheumatism and the formation of calculi. Their presence in excessive quantity aggravates all other forms of disease.

"Dr. Haig, of London, has done excellent work in the investigation of uric acid poisoning, but he becomes one-sided when he makes it the scapegoat for all disease conditions in the organism. In his philosophy of disease he fails to take into consideration the effects of other acids and systemic poisons. For instance, he does not mention the fact that carbonic acid is produced in the system somewhat similarly to the formation of coal gas in a furnace; and that its accumulation prevents the entrance of oxygen into cells and tissues, thus causing asphyxiation or oxygen starvation, which manifests in the symptoms of anaemia and tuberculosis. Neither does Dr. Haig explain the effects of other destructive by-products formed during the digestion of starches and proteins. Sulphurous acid and sulphuric acid (vitriol) as well as phosphorus and phosphoric acids actually burn up the tissues of the body. They destroy the cellulose membranes which form the protecting skins or envelopes of the cells, dissolve the protoplasm and allow the latter to escape into the circulation. This, together with pathogen obstruction, accounts for the symptoms of Bright's disease — the breaking down of the cells and the presence of albumin (cell protoplasm) in blood and urine; the clogging of the circulation; the consequent stagnation and the accumulation of blood serum (dropsy); and the final breaking down of the tissues (necrosis), resulting in open sores and ulcers.

"Excess of phosphorus and the acids from it overstimulate the brain and the nervous system, causing nervousness, irritability, hysteria and the different forms of mania. An example of this is the "distemper" of a horse when given too much oats and not enough grass or hay. The excess of phosphorus and phosphoric acids formed from the protein materials of the grain, if not neutralised by the alkaline minerals contained in grasses, hay or roots and tubers will overstimulate and irritate the nervous system of the animal and cause it to become nervous, irritable, and vicious. These symptoms disappear when the ration of oats is decreased and when more fresh grass or hay is fed in place of the grain. Hard working horses develop distemper when their food contains over five percent protein. What about inactive humans consuming much larger percentages of protein and starchy food?

"Similar effects to those produced upon the horse by an excess of grain are caused in the human organism, especially in the sensitive nervous system of the child, by a surplus of protein food, of meat, eggs, grains and pulses. Still when patients suffering from overstimulation of the brain and nervous system consult the doctor, his advice in almost every instance is: "Your nerves are weak and overwrought. You need plenty of good nourishing food (broths, meat and eggs), a good tonic and rest". The remedies prescribed by the doctor are the very things which caused the trouble in the first place."

The Relationship of Electro-Magnetically Negative Food Elements to Disease-Producing Acids, Colloids, Alkaloids and Ptomaines in the Human Body

The following diagrams plainly reveal the relationship between the electro-magnetically negative elements of the first four groups (starches, sugars, fats, proteids) and the disease-producing acids, collodis, alkaloids and ptomaines in the human body:

$$
\left.\begin{array}{l}
\text{Starches} \\
\text{Dextrins} \\
\text{Sugars} \\
\text{Fats} \\
\text{Proteids}
\end{array}\right\} \quad \begin{array}{c} \text{Composed} \\ \text{of} \\ \text{C O H N P S} \end{array}
$$

H (hydrogen) and O (oxygen) enter into the composition of the great majority of acids, alkaloids and ptomaines.

Chemical Formula	Name	
CO	Carbon monoxide	These highly poisonous gases are the products of combustion. When they accumulate in the body they cause asphyxiation, anaemia, oxygen starvation, and tuberculosis.
CO_2	Carbon dioxide carbonic acid coal gas	
$C_2H_2O_4$	Oxalic acid	These acids and their deposits in the system are responsible for headaches, catarrh, rheumatism and arthritic conditions, heart disease, arteriosclerosis, appoplexy and functional forms of diabetes and Bright's disease.
$C_5H_4N_4O_2$	Uric acid	

26

Food Elements and Disease-Producing Acids

Chemical Formula	Name
$C_4H_8O_2$	Butyric acid — forms in decaying animal matter.
H_2SO_3	Sulphurous acid (sewer gas).
H_2SO_4	Sulphuric Acid — vitriol.
H_3PO_3	Phosphorous acid.
H_3PO_4	Phosphoric acid.

The above named acids have a very irritating effect upon the organs and tissues of the body, the stronger ones being positively destructive. They must be neutralized and eliminated by the positive alkaline mineral elements of the fifth group. Meats and eggs generate in the system large amounts of these destructive acids. This explains why in spite of or rather on account of a 'highly nutritious' meat and egg diet, so many people lose flesh instead of gaining it.

Chemical Formula	Name	
$C_8H_{10}N_4O_2$	Caffeine	These alkaloids are closely related,
$C_7H_8H_4O_2$	Theobromine	chemically, to uric acid and have
$C_{10}H_{14}N_2$	Nicotine	similar effects upon the system.
C_2H_6O	Ethyl alcohol	Exists in wine, beer, whisky and other alcoholic liquors. It is formed in the digestive tract through the fermentation of sugars.

A Selection of Poisonous Ptomaines

which form in decaying animal matter and in animal and human bodies (see Chapter XVIII, "Cancer", in Volume I, *Philosophy of Natural Therapeutics*):

Chemical Formula	Name	
$C_5H_{14}N_2$	Cadaverin	Putrefying animal tissues.
$C_5H_{10}NO_2$	Cholin	Putrefying animal tissues.
$C_7H_{17}NO_2$	Gadinin	Decomposing fish.
$C_8H_{13}N$	Hydrocollidin	Decomposing fish and flesh.
CH_3N	Methylamin	Decomposing fish.
$C_5H_{13}NO$	Neurin	Putrefying flesh.
$C_{26}H_{31}NO_{17}$	Indican	A poisonous product of intestinal indigestion and putrefaction.

The foregoing substances are only a few of the dozens of different ptomaines (corpse poisons) which have been discovered in putrefying flesh and fish and in the tissues of living animal and human bodies. These morbid products of decomposing carbonaceous and protein matter form the most prolific soil for the propagation of germs, bacteria and bacilli found in typhoid fever, diphtheria, appendicitis, ptomaine poisoning, acute and chronic gastritis, enteritis, peritonitis, tuberculosis and cancer. It will be seen that all the poisonous acids, colloids, alkaloids and ptomaines mentioned are made up of the six negative, acid-forming elements (COHNPS) found in the foods of the first four groups of our classification — the starches, sugars, fats and proteins — and these poisonous by-products and end-products of starch and protein metabolism must be neutralized and eliminated from the system by the positive alkaline mineral elements which abound in the food materials of the fifth group, especially in the juicy fruits and vegetables.

These facts in nature form the scientific basis of Natural Dietetics and rational vegetarianism as well as of the philosophy and practice of Natural Therapeutics. That they are "facts in nature" has been proved by the investigators of the vitamins as shown in a later chapter.

CHAPTER VI

THE TENSING AND RELAXING EFFECTS OF FOODS UPON THE DIGESTIVE ORGANS AND THE SYSTEM AS A WHOLE

There are two forces at work in the human organism, the one tensing and contracting, the other relaxing and expanding. Normal function, or health, results from equilibrium between the two. The equilibrium between contending forces we call the positive condition of health; departure from it in either direction, the negative condition of disease. As a rule acids exert a tensing, contracting influence, alkalis relax and expand. These facts should be kept in mind when studying the physiology and psychology of foods and medicines.

The extremes of tension and relaxation are expressed in the functions of the body by constipation and diarrhoea. We find that as a rule, acid or acid producing foods have a contracting, constipating influence and alkaline foods a relaxing laxative influence. If the intestines are functioning normally, the faeces should pass freely and easily; they should be well formed and leave the parts perfectly clean. After an evacuation there should be a feeling of perfect cleanliness, of freedom and of buoyancy. It is possible to have daily passages from the intestines and yet to retain hard incrustations of foetid matter. A person may suffer from malnutrition, deficient elimination and autointoxication because the faeces are unable to force a passage through hardened accumulations. Often this condition is indicated by the thinness of the discharges. If the faeces are black, too much of the bile and uric acid producing foods (proteins) have been taken. If they are too light, probably not enough proteins and starches are consumed.

The extremes of tension are illustrated, on the one hand by the collaemic forms of uric acid poisoning, in which the capillaries are blocked, surface circulation impeded, blood in the arteries and vital organs at high tension, bowels sluggish and constipated; on the other hand, the extremes of relaxation are characterized by weakened blood vessels and flabby muscles. The blood serum seems to leak in morbid perspiration from the relaxed tissues, and the bowels are usually very loose.

In mental and psychic conditions, the extreme of tension is portrayed in the excitable, overactive, talkative, boisterous and sometimes violent types of nervousness, hysteria and delusional insanity. The extreme of relaxation is exhibited in weak, negative, psychic cases. These patients are languid, listless, indifferent to surroundings, too apathetic to eat, dress or attend to their bodily needs.

Proteins   (Group IV)

We have seen that protein materials are made up of six negative acid producing elements (COHNPS). Proteins are, therefore, above all others, acid producing foods. In the metabolism of the body they produce uric, carbonic, sulphuric, phosphoric, oxalic and a number of other acids; therefore, it is not surprising that protein foods are constipating. Lean meats, fish and fowl, if taken by themselves, are very constipating. Fat meats, taken in moderation and in right combinations, have a lubricating, laxative effect; if taken in excess they produce constipation and a sticky condition of the bowels and faeces; eggs, being rich in albumen, sulphur and phosphorus, when taken by themselves or in combination with other tensing foods, are also constipating. Milk in small quantities has, for many, a constipating effect; taken in large quantities it often has a laxative effect, because of the amount of water with which the system is deluged; in other cases, existing constipation is intensified by this practice.

The vegetable products richest in protein are the legumes (peas, beans and lentils) and the cereals. These are generally called the glutenous or nitrogenous foods. If taken by themselves or in combination with other tensing foods they have a constipating effect; the faeces become hard and brittle. Nuts, being rich in fats and proteid, if taken in excess or with other tensing foods, also have a constipating effect.

Carbohydrates   (Groups I and II)

Foods belonging to the carbohydrate groups, which in the natural state occur in combination with large amounts of organic salts and other laxative principles, do not impede the normal activities of the intestines, unless taken in excess. Such foods are whole grain preparations of cereals and the unrefined brown sugar products of cane, beet and maple. The starchy and glutenous principles of the pure cane sugar, when artificially extracted from natural food products, become proximate and inorganic food elements, which, separated from the organic salt and other laxative principles, exert a tensing and constipating influence. Such proximate food elements are starch, gluten, white sugar, and the like. Honey is one of nature's finest foods. Besides being rich in saccharin matter it contains positive mineral elements and is animated with the animal life element. Molasses is much more laxative than white sugar, because it contains the organic salts of which the refined sugar has been robbed.

Hydrocarbons   (Group III)

Animal fats, cream and vegetable oils, taken in moderation, have a purely mechanical laxative effect, because they act as lubricators to the organism as a whole and especially to the intestinal tract. If taken in excess, however, or in combination with tensing foods, they have a constipating effect, because the liver and pancreas cannot furnish sufficient amounts of bile and steapsin for their reduction, and fats which fail to be reduced or saponified produce a sticky condition of the intestines. Even too much olive oil, which many vegetarians seem to think can be taken without harm, may, therefore, become a source of constipation. We must not overlook the fact that it is a proximate element. The olive itself, containing the oily principles in combination with moderate percentages of organic salts, has a much more beneficial effect.

Organic Salts   (Group V)

In this group belong all foods comparatively poor in proteins, carbohydrates and hydrocarbons, and rich in the organic salts of sodium, iron, lime, magnesium and potassium. The most valuable in this respect are the green, leafy vegetables such as spinach, lettuce, cabbage, celery, kale, asparagus, watercress, the green tops of roots, and so on. Next in order come the roots: radishes, carrots, parsnips, beets, swedes, onions and horseradish. Potatoes, although they contain considerable amounts of potassium and lime, are deficient in sodium, iron and magnesium. However, they are rich in bone building minerals and vitamins. On the whole, the starchy elements predominate over the organic salts and they are, therefore, placed in the carbohydrate group. Among the fruits, the banana corresponds to the potato; it is rich in starchy and saccharin elements, but comparatively poor in organic salts.

Nature's Wise Provision

It is interesting to note how, for each season of the year, nature furnishes the foods and medicines best adapted to changing conditions. In the fall we gather the hardy, nourishing, heat and energy producing cereals, legumes and nuts, which furnish the fuel materials necessary to do the winter's work and to protect us against cold. These acid-producing foods, through their tensing contracting influences, help us to retain the heat of the body; on the other hand they also favour the retention of waste matter and poisons. During the winter season the accumulation of fermentable waste matter in the system is brought on by increased amounts of food, closed doors and windows and pores contracted and closed by the cold. With the first thaws of springtime these waste materials begin to ferment and to produce fevers, colds and catarrhs. Nature again provides the proper foods and remedies: lettuce, spinach, young onions, watercress, rhubarb, asparagus, and other tender, luscious vegetables. These furnish the best laxatives and diuretics — those which most effectively assist nature in her spring house cleaning. In the heat of summer the watery, refreshing and cooling melons, cantaloups and cucumbers are the most effective agents in relaxing the bowels and the pores of the skin, allowing free evacuation and increasing heat evaporation through the surface of the body. These delicious summer foods owe their relaxing qualities to the large percentage of alkaline salts which they contain. Their purging effect need not be feared. By cleansing the system of waste matter and poisons this purging prevents dangerous inflammations and fevers.

CHAPTER VII

STANDARD FOODS

Milk and Arterial Blood the only Standard Food Combinations in Nature

Animal and human bodies are composed of certain well defined elements, in certain well defined proportions. Chemistry so far has discovered seventeen of these elements in appreciable quantities and ascertained their more important functions in the body. If any of these are present in over abundance, and others are deficient in quantity or wholly lacking, there will be abnormal function, or disease. Therefore, the elements of nutrition must be provided in right proportions in order to meet the needs of the body. The quest of natural food reformers after a normal, natural diet is hence not so silly and impossible as some people would have us believe. Many old school food scientists, also, have recognized the desirability and possibility of establishing standard food combinations. But all these authorities, whether they are advocates of the meat, mixed, or vegetarian diet, deal only with proteins, fats and carbohydrates. This is shown by the "Standard Daily Rations" which appear in most medical text books which are used in universities and medical schools. In these books the diet which is recommended as "normal" should consist of 100 to 120 grams of proteins, 90 to 100 grams of fats, and 250 to 333 grams of carbohydrates. The nutritive value of a diet is said to depend chiefly upon the amount of carbon and nitrogen it contains, which implies that protein and carbohydrate foods are the most important.[1]

The leaders of American vegetarianism, building on these old school theories and food standards in making up their vegetarian diet combinations, searched principally for substitutes for meat and eggs, that is, for foods rich in proteins, fats and starches. As a consequence, we find that the dietetics of our best known vegetarian sanatoriums and food reformers deal mainly with proteins, fats and carbohydrates. The daily bulletins giving dietary advice to the patients of these institutions deal with these, the proximate food elements only.

---

[1]
The number of elements to be found in the body by scientific analysis has now been shown to be considerably greater than seventeen and a certain amount of knowledge has been accumulated on the functions performed in the body by the small amounts of certain elements which appear to be essential to the body economy. However, it should not be assumed that all elements of which traces are commonly found in the body are necessary to its proper functioning. Some of them may be unnecessary or even positively harmful.

All widely advertised breakfast and predigested health foods in the market are made up of grains, peas, beans, peanuts, cocoa-nuts or combinations of these food materials. Breaking up these natural products of the soil into proximate elements, such as protose, gluten, white flour, white sugar, and the like, and devitalizing them by cooking, steaming and roasting tends to make them more negative than they were in the natural state. The proximate elements, proteins, fats and carbohydrates dealt with in old school dietetics, contain six elements only out of the seventeen found in the human body. What about the others, the mineral elements? All the "regular" authorities merely mention these all-important mineral elements and bunch them as "inorganic salts" or "ash", and claim that any adequate food supply of proteins, fats and carbohydrates carries enough of these "inorganic salts" to satisfy the needs of the body. This assumption, however, is superficial, and altogether unscientific. We shall prove in these pages, and by means of tabulated analyses, that exactly the reverse is true — that the organic salts or mineral elements are of the greatest importance in the vital functions of the body; that the only danger lies in the excessive use of proteins, fats and carbohydrates; and that the difficulty in rational dietetics lies in procuring in the daily dietary a sufficient amount of organic mineral salts without at the same time overloading the system with starchy and nitrogenous elements.

The authorities also make a mistake in stating their normal diet combinations in weight. This is always misleading, as the amount of food needed by different individuals differs very much in weight. Stuffing food into patients by weight in accordance with "standard rations" has stuffed numbers of them into early graves. An amount of food in weight just sufficient for the needs of one person may prove altogether too much for the next one. The only rational way to calculate food proportions is by percentages. In order to accomplish this readily it is necessary to establish a standard combination of food elements in such proportions or percentages as will meet all requirements of the human organism. Milk was selected by some German scientists as such a standard food combination because nature made it a perfect food for the new-born and growing animal, and because it is capable of sustaining the growing organism in perfect health and strength. Furthermore, the analyses of Dr. Lahman and other chemists disclose the interesting fact that the elementary composition of the milk of an animal is just about the same as the ash of its body after cremation. Milk is, indeed, a perfect food for the growing animal, but it is not so to be considered for the adult animal or man. The reason for this is that the young and growing animal requires a great deal more of potassium and calcium, the tissue building elements, than the full grown adult body. On the other hand, the young animal, on account of its greater elasticity, plasticity, and natural activity in play and sports, eliminates waste matter much more readily, and, therefore, needs less of the eliminative elements than the mature body. This is indicated by a comparison of the analyses of blood and milk. While milk is richer in the building elements, the blood of the adult animal is richer in sodium and iron, the positive "working" elements.[2]

[2]
    Lindlahr believed that a "natural" and healthy diet was the most important single factor in producing and maintaining health and that it was an easy matter to work out and to follow such a diet in a rational and scientific way. As he expresses it, "there can and must be a combination of food elements which in certain well defined proportions will fit the demands of the normal human body". He gave a number of definitions of natural food and natural diet and worked out a system by which all common foods can be classified in accordance with their chemical composition and their nutritional function in the body. In defining what is "natural" food he says that it is "that food which appeals to the senses of sight, taste and smell in the natural condition as it comes from nature's hands". For making up a "natural diet" he gives a number of instructions. "A rational vegetarian diet properly combined, consisting of dairy products, the positive vegetables and fruits and just enough of starchy and protein foods to supply the needs of the body for tissue building and fuel material, will be found sufficient to keep people in health and strength in the most trying circumstances. It is sufficient if a fair proportion, say one half, of a meal consists of raw food and the other half of cooked food." To make use of his system of food classification he says that "a natural diet which is to fill the demands of the human organism must consist of one half of the food materials of Group V (mineral elements) and one half of the food elements of Groups I, II, III and IV (starches, sugars, fats and proteins). Any meal or diet composed in those proportions conforms to what we designate as normal or natural in food combinations". Another test of a diet being "natural" is that in its component elements it conforms to the chemical composition of milk or red (arterial) blood which should be regarded as standards of what the body requires in the right proportions, From this it will be seen that Lindlahr regards a good and healthy diet as being a matter of proportions and not a matter of amounts or of calories, nearly all diets now in common use having a sufficiency or too much of carbohydrates and proteins but an insufficiency of positive mineral elements. Since Lindlahr's time the movement for diet reform has acquired a considerable momentum though it has not as yet invaded the medical profession or its dieticians to the extent which might be expected or is desirable. However, there are signs that a change is coming in dietetic thought and practice, much of it in line with Lindlahr's ideas. For instance, the importance of having a proportion of uncooked food and foods which provide roughage and vitamins is now very generally recognized. There is also beginning to be a realization of the dangers of additives, preservatives and colouring matters in foods, of the undesirability of the present enormous consumption of tea, coffee, alcoholic beverages, fats and meat, and the harmfulness of denatured and refined sugar and flour. In this connection it is of interest to note that there is not very much difference between the kind of diet advocated by Lindlahr and that which is recommended by the McCarrison Society and set forth in Dr. James Lambert Mount's book, "The Food and Health of Western Man".

Dietetics in a Nutshell

Food Classes	Predominant Chemical Elements	Functions in Vital Processes	Foods in which the Elements of the Respective Groups Predominate
GROUP I Carbohydrates — Starches	Carbon Oxygen Hydrogen	Producers of Heat and Energy	**Cereals:** The inner, white parts of wheat, corn, rye, oats, barley, buckwheat and rice **Vegetables:** Potatoes, roots, sweet potatoes, pumpkins, squashes **Fruits:** Bananas **Nuts:** Chestnuts
GROUP II Carbohydrates — Dextrins and Sugars	Carbon Oxygen Hydrogen	Producers of Heat and Energy	**Vegetables:** Melons, beets, sorghum **Fruits:** Bananas, dates, figs, grapes, raisins **Dairy Products:** Milk **Natural Sugars:** Honey, maple sugar **Commercial Sugars:** White sugar, syrup. glucose, candy **Nuts:** Cocoa-nuts
GROUP III Fats — Fats and Oils	Carbon Oxygen Hydrogen	Producers of Heat and Energy	**Fruits:** Olives **Dairy Products:** Cream, butter, cheese **Nuts:** Peanuts, almonds, walnuts, cocoa-nuts, Brazil nuts, pecans, pignolias, etc **Commercial Fats:** Olive oil, peanut oil, peanut butter, vegetable cooking oils **The yolks of eggs**
GROUP IV Proteins — Albumen (white of egg) Gluten (grains) Myosin (lean meat)	Carbon Oxygen Hydrogen Nitrogen Phosphorus Sulphur	Producers of Heat and Energy Building and Repair Materials for Cells and Tissues	**Cereals:** The outer, dark parts of wheat, corn, rye, oats, barley, buckwheat and rice **Vegetables:** The legumes (peas, beans, lentils), mushrooms **Nuts:** Cocoa-nuts, chestnuts, peanuts, pignolias (pine nuts), hickory nuts, hazelnuts, walnuts, pecans, etc. **Diary Products:** Milk, cheese **Meats:** Muscular parts of animals, fish and fowl.
GROUP V Organic Minerals — Organic Mineral Elements	Sodium, Na Ferrum, Fe Calcium, Ca Potassium, K Magnesium, Mg Manganese, Mn Silicon, Si Chlorine, Cl Fluorine, F	Eliminators, Blood, bone and nerve builders; Antiseptics; Blood purifiers; Laxatives; Cholagogues; Producers of electro-magnetic energies	**The red blood of animals.** **Cereals:** The hulls and outer, dark layers of grains and rice **Vegetables:** Lettuce, spinach, cabbage, green peppers, watercress, celery, onions, asparagus, cauliflower, tomatoes, stringbeans, fresh peas, parsley, cucumbers, radishes, savoy, horseradish, dandelions, beets, carrots, turnips, salsify, artichokes, leek, Brussels sprouts, parsnips, squashes, sorghum, kohlrabi, eggplant **Fruits:** Apples, pears, peaches, oranges, lemons, grapefruit, plums, prunes, cranberries, raspberries, gooseberries, currants **Dairy Products:** Milk, buttermilk, skimmed milk **Nuts:** Cocoa-nuts

35

CHAPTER VIII

DIGESTION AND ASSIMILATION

Digestion and assimilation may be divided into the following stages:
1. Intake of Food;
2. Mastication;
3. Insalivation;
4. Deglutition;
5. Chymification in the stomach;
6. Chylification through intestinal digestion;
7. Absorption of the chyle by the membrances lining the intestinal tract, and its transmission through the lacteal and venous vessels into the circulation;
8. Elimination and defaecation of the end-products and waste materials of digestion.

The limited space of this volume does not admit of going into the details of the various processes. They can be studied in any encyclopaedia or work on physiology. We shall confine ourselves to giving a brief outline of the processes of digestion and assimilation in so far as this will facilitate a better understanding of the problems of Natural Dietetics discussed in this volume.

The office of digestion is to prepare the foodstuffs for absorption into the fluids of the body, and for utilization in the various processes of nutrition. To make this possible, the coarse and complex food materials have to be dissolved and rendered diffusible in order to facilitate their absorption through the membranes of the epithelial cells which cover the walls of the intestinal tract. This breaking up of the complex food materials into simpler compounds, or into their constituent, proximate elements is accomplished by the influence of the digestive ferments secreted by the microzymes in the cells of certain glandular structures belonging to the digestive apparatus.

In the following brief survey of the processes of digestion and assimilation, we shall follow the various food materials through their transformations to their final destination in the vital economy of the body. Orthodox physiology and food chemistry, as we have pointed out, deal with three food classes only. These are: (1) the carbohydrates, comprising starches, dextrins and sugars; (2) the hydrocarbons, comprising fats and oils; (3) proteins, the principal representatives of which are albumen (white of egg), gluten of grains and legumes, myosin of fleshy tissues, serum-globulin of the blood, haemoglobin of the red blood corpuscles, lactalbumin and casein of milk and cheese.

Digestion of Starches

The starches are acted on in the mouth, after thorough mastication and insalivation, by the ferment ptyalin of the saliva, and transformed into dextrins and sugars (maltose and glucose). Ptyalin acts only in an alkaline or neutral medium. If the starches are thoroughly masticated and insalivated, the action of the ptyalin continues for twenty to forty minutes in the stomach. By that time its action is checked by the acidity of the gastric juices. The transformation of the starches (after they leave the stomach) into the simplest and most refined forms of dextroses and glucoses (sugars) continues in the intestines under the influence of the pancreatic ferment amylase or amylopsin. The ferment, invertase, found in the intestinal fluid, changes cane sugar into levulose, and the latter into glucose. The starches must be reduced to dextroses and glucoses before they can be assimilated by the epithelial cells lining the intestinal walls and before they can be transmitted through these into the circulation.

From what has been said it becomes apparent why it is necessary thoroughly to masticate and insalivate all starchy foods. This is of especial importance for those who suffer from intestinal indigestion. If starchy foods, as is usually done, are made slippery with milk and cream and swallowed down without being thoroughly mixed with saliva, they remain unchanged in their passage through mouth and stomach. If there is a tendency towards, or actual condition of intestinal indigestion, the starches are not transformed at all, and instead of being absorbed into the circulation as valuable fuel materials in the forms of dextroses and glucoses, they enter into processes of decay and fermentation, filling the system with noxious gases and poisons. If more starchy food materials are taken in than can be absorbed by the circulation and utilized by cells and tissues, part of the surplus is stored in the liver and in the muscles in the form of glycogen, to be drawn upon when the intake of carbohydrates falls below the requirements of the body. In Chapter III we have described Dr. Thomas Powell's ingenious and plausible theory of the conversion of the carbon compounds in the cells of the muscles and other tissues of the body into heat and muscular energy.

Digestion of Fats

The fats are not acted on at all by the saliva and by the gastric juice of the stomach, only in so far as the hydrochloric acid of the latter partly digests and dissolves the membranes of the fat globules, rendering their contents more soluble and more prone to the action of the fat splitting ferments in the intestinal tract. The principal one of these ferments is the lipase (steapsin) of the pancreatic fluid. The action of the lipase is greatly facilitated and intensified by the bile. In fact, the digestive activity of all the pancreatic ferments becomes possible only after the contents of the intestinal tract (chyme and chyle) have been changed from the acid condition, in which they left the stomach, to the alkaline, because the pancreatic and intestinal ferments act in an alkaline medium only.

The fats are split up into glycerin and fatty acids. These end-products of fatty digestion are absorbed by the epithelial cells lining the intestinal walls. While passing through these cells the glycerin and fatty acids are reunited and built up into fat globules, and these are transmitted through the lacteal vessels into the lymphatic circulation, and finally into the venous circulation, to be further refined and prepared for assimilation, in their passage through the liver.

Digestion of the Proteins

Protein food materials serve two principal purposes. They are composed of six elements (COHNPS). The first three elements may be used in the economy of the body for the production of heat and energy, in the same way as the (COH) molecules in carbohydrates and hydrocarbons, but aside from this the proteid food materials serve other important purposes in the building up and repairing of cells and tissues. The substance of cells consists of protoplasm, that is, protein matter; therefore, the building and repair of cells requires protein foodstuffs. But the transformation of the protein materials as they exist in foods into protein substances of the living cells and tissues of the human body involves profound changes, different from and far more complex than the simple hydrolytic reduction of carbohydrates and hydrocarbons.

The progressive digestive changes of the proteins into proteose, peptones and amino-acids begin in the stomach under the influence of the pepsin secreted by the cell linings of the stomach. The pepsin acts only in an acid medium and this is created by the hydrochloric acid which forms part of the gastric secretions. The transformation of the proteins continues in the intestinal tract under the action of the trypsin. The trypsin is not, as was formerly believed, solely a secretion of the pancreas, but is in reality a compound formed by the chemical union of trypsinogen of the pancreatic fluid with enterokinase secreted by the epithelial cells of the intestinal walls, especially in the duodenum. The trypsin acts only in an alkaline medium, and this is furnished by the inpouring of the bile into the chyme as the latter enters the intestines in its periodic discharges from the stomach. It seems to be the acidity of the chyme and the ferment secretions of the pancreatic juice, as well as the secretion of the enterokinase, which stimulate the flow of the bile into the duodenum. The transformation of protein food materials into proteose, peptones and amino-acids continues in the intestines, and these refined forms of protein matter are then absorbed by the cell lining of the intestinal walls and elaborated into the more complex protein substances as they exist in the human body.

The Processes of Digestion

The following diagram presents in concise form a survey of the most important phases of digestion.

Food Products	Acted Upon By	Changed Into	Serve As
Starch	The ptyalin of the saliva in the mouth and stomach. The amylase of the intestinal fluids.	Dextrins Dextrose Maltose Glucose	
Cane Sugar	Invertase of the intestinal fluids	Levulose and this into Glucose	Fuel materials and producers of muscular energy
Milk	Rennin of the stomach. Lactase of the intestinal fluids	Changes milk sugar into galactose and this into Glucose	
Fats	1. Hydrochloric acid of the stomach 2. Bile of liver and lipase of pancreatic fluid.	1. Digests cell membranes of fat globules 2. Change fats into glycerin and fatty acids	
Proteins Albumen Serum-globulin Haemoglobin Myosinogen Gluten	Pepsin of stomach and trypsin of intestinal fluid. Trypsin is composed of the trypsinogen of the pancreatic fluid in combination with the enterokinase of the intestinal fluid	Changes proteins into proteose, peptones and amino-acids	Producers of heat and energy. Building and repair materials for the cells and tissues of the body.

To recapitulate, the breaking down of all food materials into simpler and more refined compounds serves several purposes:

(1) to separate waste and indigestible matter from the nutritious substances;

(2) to make food materials sufficiently soluble and diffusible so that they can be assimilated by the absorbent membranes of the intestinal tract;

(3) to liberate their latent heat and vital energy;

(4) to change the coarse compounds of food materials into the more refined and complex materials of the living cells and tissues of the human body.

If we assimilated animal blood, flesh and fat in their original forms the tissues of our bodies would soon resemble those of pigs, cows and sheep. In order to preserve the individuality and integrity of the various species and families of animals and of man, it is necessary that all food materials be broken down first into their simplest compounds and proximate elements and then reconstructed (synthetized) into the building materials, cells, tissues and organs of the animal or human being which consumes the foods.

CHAPTER IX

THE TRUE NATURE AND SOURCE OF VITAMINS OR LIFE ELEMENTS

The opening paragraphs and later passages of this treatise on vitamins may impress the reader more like a sermon than a scientific essay on food values. This is not at all unusual or unreasonable. Science is rapidly becoming more religious and religion more scientific. The laws and principles underlying the science of dietetics and the art of healing human ailments cannot be comprehended and applied without an understanding of the psychical and spiritual basis of physical material things and forces. The greatest of all gifts bestowed upon us by Cosmic, Creative Intelligence is life. Upon this primary gift of all gifts depend consciousness, individual intelligence, reason, creative will, and all else. More life means better health, more strength, greater efficiency in the business of life, increased capacity for loving and serving, and therefore greater happiness. "That sounds beautiful and true," you say, "but how can we receive more life when we cannot create it, when we do not know what it is?" What about electricity? Ask Edison, Marconi, or any other great electrician, what this mysterious force is. They will tell you: "We do not know." Yet they have harnessed the lightning to their machines and made it our obedient servant. So it is with vital force. We cannot create it; we do not know what it is. If we did, we would know God; we would know all there is to be known in this universe. However, we do know this primary force of all forces through its manifestations in living bodies, and by complying with the laws and principles which govern its phenomena, we can open ourselves to a more abundant inflow of vital energy.

This is what the Master meant when he said: "I am come that they might have life, and that they might have it more abundantly." In these words the Master, Jesus, not only gave us the formula for the healing of human ailments and for the expression of the highest possible degree of efficiency on the physical, mental, moral and spiritual planes of being, but He also disclosed the principle underlying the evolutionary development of the sidereal universe, from the tiniest atom of matter to the greatest solar system. Evolutionary development means the manifestation and expression of more life in ever-increasing degrees of potency, refinement and complexity. How did the Master, Jesus, fulfill his promise? By feeding his followers plenty of rich and nourishing food? By giving them poisonous tonics and stimulants? No, he taught them how to comply with the higher laws of their being, how to become more perfect in body, mind and soul, and in that way to open themselves to a more abundant inflow of life and vital energy.[1]

Weak, sick humanity cries out in despair: "Oh doctor, if you could only prescribe some nourishing food or tonic to give me more strength, then I would be all right". Through all the ages, alchemists, doctors and scientists have been searching in vain for the wonderful elixir which will rejuvenate the body, cure all human ills and prolong human life indefinitely, and indeed we would be able to cure all disease instantaneously if we could sufficiently increase the inflow and activity of vital energy. All disease is caused by something that interferes with, diminishes or disturbs the normal inflow and distribution of vital energy throughout the system. Vigour, physical and mental, power of resistance to disease, and capacity of enjoyment of life are manifestations of vital energy and these are transmutations of vital force. The

[1]
    Though Jesus Christ, according to the four gospels, was a great healer of the sick it is somewhat remarkable that Christianity in the form in which it has developed and been taught and handed down in the western world has, unlike other great religions, very little to say about how people should feed and look after their bodies. There is some evidence that this was not always so. The so-called Gospel of Peace of Jesus Christ which has been studied and translated from the original Aramaic by Edmond Szekely and Purcell Weaver (published by the C.W. Daniel Co) would seem to throw a new and different light on Jesus Christ and the Christian message from that which is to be derived from the four gospels as we now know them.

problem, then, before us in the healing of disease as well as in maintaining the greatest possible efficiency and capacity for enjoyment of the finer pleasures of life, is to increase the inflow and distribution of life force — which means "life more abundant". This glorious consummation has been and always will be out of reach so long as the medical profession and laity look for the source of vital energy in "nourishing foods and strengthening tonics and stimulants." These substances cannot bestow life, because they are secondary manifestations of life. Secondary, derived energies cannot be transmuted back into life force — the primary source of all kinds of energy. If this were possible, we could, indeed, prolong life indefinitely.

We hear you say: "If this were true, why do we have to eat and drink to keep alive?" "Why do we waste away and die when we abstain from food and drink?" This is the answer. All that food and drink can do is to keep the organism in the right condition so that vital force can manifest and operate through it to the best advantage. To this end food is needed to build up and repair the cells and tissues of the body. It also serves to a certain extent as fuel material which is transmuted into animal heat and energy. But this does not account for the enormous amount of animal heat and energy constantly liberated and expended by the animal or human body. Just as coal has to come in touch with fire before it can be transmuted into heat, so the life force is needed to "burn up" or "explode" the fuel materials in the body. When "Life" has departed, even large amounts of sugars, fats, proteins, tonics and stimulants are not able to produce one spark of vital energy in the dead body. Instead of increasing vital energy, overeating wastes it. Digestion and assimilation of food and drink and elimination of waste materials require the expenditure of considerable amounts of vital energy. Therefore, all food taken in excess of the actual needs of the body wastes vital force instead of giving it. If these facts were more generally known and appreciated, people would not habitually overeat under the mistaken idea that their vitality increases in proportion to the amount of food they consume; neither would they believe that they can derive strength from poisonous stimulants and tonics. They would not be so much afraid of fasting. They would understand better the necessity of fasting in acute diseases and healing crises and avail themselves more frequently of this most effective means of purification. They would no longer believe themselves in danger of dying if they were to miss a few meals.

Nothing has proved more positively the fact that there must be another source of animal heat and energy besides food and drink, than the long fasts frequently undergone for therapeutic and other purposes.

42

Since Dr. Tanner completed his forty-day fast, fasting has become popular as one of the best methods of physical, mental and moral regeneration. During the last eighteen years hundreds of people have fasted under our observation and direction. These fasts were continued from a few days to six weeks; in several cases as long as seven weeks. These long fasts did not prove harmful in any way, but on the contrary they resulted in improved health and were followed in time by gains in flesh and strength.

As long as reports of long fasts and their beneficial effects come from physicians advocating drugless healing methods, the veracity of these accounts may be questioned by the medical profession and the laity, but at the present time proof of the possibility of such long extended fasts comes from an unexpected source. To quote from a pamphlet the writer issued near the climax of the fasting protest in Ireland: "It is now ninety-one days, or thirteen weeks, since the Irish hunger strikers started on their long martyrdom. During the first few weeks of their fasting, I predicted that they could go ten weeks without food before reaching the danger point. This proved true. Of the eleven confined in the Cork prison, Fitzgerald was the first to die, on the seventy-second day of his fast. MacSwiney began to have fainting spells on the seventy-first day of his fast. The attending physicians started to feed him while temporarily unconscious. During his waking moments, however, he vigourously resisted it. This martyr to the cause of his beloved country passed away on the seventy-fourth day. He would have lived longer if beef juice and alcoholic stimulants, two of the worst things on which to break a fast, had not been forced upon him. The daily papers stated that during the last few days of his life his temperature was normal. At the time of this writing the eleven hunger strikers in Cork prison have completed their thirteenth week. The temperature of their bodies is still near normal or only a few degrees below." If food and drink, as claimed by the medical profession and materialistic scientists in general, is the only source of animal heat and energy, why is it that the temperature in those starving bodies remains near normal to the very end, when all the reserves of nourishing substances have become exhausted, when nothing is left of their wasted bodies but skin and bones? If the mechanistic theory of vital force is true, if human bodies depend for heat and energy on food and drink like the boiler on the coal which is shovelled into the furnace, why is it that the temperature in those starving bodies towards the end did not gradually decline? Why did it keep above ninety degrees to the last breath and then drop suddenly to the temperature of the surrounding atmosphere? What is it that keeps the heat in those bodies up to normal after all fuel materials have been exhausted? The only possible explanation is that there must be another source of heat and energy besides food and drink and the reserve stores of flesh and fat in the body. Think of the enormous amount of heat and energy liberated and expended by a body in normal health during twenty-four hours. Not long ago a prominent authority made the statement that it had been proved by scientific experiments that the amount of power necessary to draw one full breath was equal to an amount of energy required to lift a five hundred pound weight two inches from the floor. If this is true, what immense amounts of energy must be required to perform the thousands of different forms of physical, chemical, mental and emotional activities going on in the living human body every moment of its existence.

We do not know whether the statement before alluded to is true or not. We do know, however, that very large amounts of energy must be required to expand the breathing apparatus with its heavy and complicated mass of bones, ligaments and muscles, to force the large amount of blood through the arteries and capillaries of the body against resistance, besides hundreds of other forms of working energy continuously active during waking and sleeping hours. In addition to this, imagine the enormous amount of heat necessary to keep a full-grown human body up to normal temperature during twenty-four hours. The totals of heat and energy thus liberated and expended must amount to an equivalent of thousands of pounds of steam. Does anyone of sane mind believe that this enormous amount of heat and working energy can be derived from a few pounds of food and drink consumed by a human being in the course of a day? Still this is boldly claimed by exponents of the materialistic or mechanistic theory of life and vital energy. It is the basis of the caloric theory of food values.

As before stated, all that food and drink can do is to keep the body in normal, healthy condition. On this depends the flow of life force into the body and its free distribution by way of the sympathetic and central nervous systems to the various organs and to every individual cell. Anything and everything in natural methods of living and treatment that will help to nourish and purify the blood, that will rid the system of waste and morbid matter, that will correct mechanical lesions and harmonize mental and emotional conditions will ensure a greater supply of life force and its derivatives — strength, vitality, resistance, and recuperative power. In other words, the more normal, healthy and perfect the organism, the more copious will be the inflow of vital energy.

All the different schools, systems, and cults of healing deal only in a partial way with the problems of vital force. Some confine their efforts to dietetic measures, others to administration of drugs and to surgical treatment. The hydropath stimulates the flow of vital fluids and nerve currents through hot and cold water applications. Manipulative schools of healing endeavour to facilitate the distribution of vital energy through the system by correcting mechanical lesions in the bony structures, ligaments, muscles and connective tissues. Mental scientists, Christian Scientists, and spiritual healers confine their efforts to establishing the right mental and spiritual attitude. All these and other systems of treating human ailments deal only with one or several phases of the problem. The only system which endeavours to combine and apply all that is good in natural healing methods is Nature Cure. It draws the line only at the employment of destructive methods, such as the use of poisonous drugs, filthy disease products, promiscuous, uncalled for surgical operations, hypnotism and mental therapeutics based on erroneous and misleading premises.

CHAPTER X

WHO DISCOVERED THE VITAMINS OR LIFE ELEMENTS?

Nothing in the field of dietetics has created such widespread and genuine interest as the "discovery of vitamins". It is true that the vitamins are of primary importance in the processes of nutrition, but are they a "new discovery"? The word "vitamin" means "life substance" or "life element", and we have talked about the life element in foods ever since we began to lecture and to write on natural dietetics. The term, life elements, as far as we know, was first used by Florence Huntley in *Harmonies of Evolution*. One of the first articles dealing with the subject of vitamins, under that name, appeared in the Britannica Year Book for 1913. It was entitled *Cause and Cure of Beriberi*, was written by Dr. Paget and reads as follows:

"In 1909 Fraser and Stanton published their *Aetiology of Beriberi*. Working on lines suggested by C. Hose and Braddon, they traced the cause of the disease to the use of "milled" rice, i.e. rice which has been "polished" by the removal of its husk and outer layers. Fowls or pigeons fed on polished rice alone quickly showed signs of the disease; but if the polishings of the rice were added to their food they quickly recovered. Further observations by De Hann, Chamberlain, Eijkmann, and others showed that the disease was not due simply to the absence of phosphates from the rice. It was due to the loss of a substance which is present as a mere trace in the husks; indeed, there are no more than ten grains of it in a ton of rice. Funk, working at the Lister Institute, has lately segregated this substance, and has given it the name of "vitamin". The wonder does not end here for Funk also isolated from limes a substance similar to "vitamin" and present in about one in 100,000 parts of the fruit. This "vitamin" of the lime has a favourable action alike on beriberi and on scurvy".

Since Dr. Paget, Casimir Funk and others first used the term "vitamin", much has been said and written about this interesting subject, but nowhere outside of our own writings has an explanation been offered as to what these mysterious substances or forces really are. As before stated, for the last eighteen years we have been writing and talking about the existence and functions of the *life elements* in foods—and the *life elements* are identical with the *vitamins*. It is, to say the least, a curious coincidence that the word "vitamin" is a literal translation of the term "life element" which we have been using to denote the manifestations and activities of the life force in foods and living bodies. In the November, 1908, issue of the *Nature Cure Magazine*, we wrote about the life elements as follows:

"In every higher kingdom of nature, matter is made to vibrate to higher ratios of vibratory motion and moulded into compounds of increasing complexity and of greater refinement of texture. Four distinct life elements, or "ranges of vibration", control the four great kingdoms of life on this earth plane. These life elements are manifestations of life force in physical, chemical, mental, emotional, spiritual and psychical activities. The lowest or mineral plane is controlled by the electro-magnetic life element; the next higher or vegetable kingdom by the vito-chemical life element; the still higher animal kingdom is animated by the spiritual or animal life element; and the highest or human plane by the soul or psychical life element.

In the mineral kingdom the electro-magnetic life element binds together by chemical affinity the atoms into the simple inorganic compounds of the mineral plane. In the vegetable kingdom, the vito-chemical life elements, by the aid of sun heat and energy, builds up the simple compounds of earthy elements, air and water, into the refined and complex living molecules of organic vegetable matter. The elements of earth, air, sun heat and water, thus organized or made alive in the vegetable cell by the vitochemical life element, furnish the foods for the next higher animal and human planes. The animal life element governing the animal kingdom seizes upon the living matter of the vegetable plane and refines, organizes and vivifies it to still higher potencies of vital force and creative energy and introduces the psychical elements of consciousness, instinctive intelligence and volition. The human kingdom is animated by the soul or psychic life element. Under its influence animal consciousness matures into human self consciousness; instinctive intelligence and volition develop into human reason, will power and self control.

To recapitulate: The four great kingdoms of earth life are animated and governed by four distinct life elements which are equivalent to progressively higher and more refined ranges of vibratory activity, and increase of vibratory activity means increase of kinetic or working energy. These facts in natural science explain why, in every higher kingdom, molecules become more complex, and possessed of greater potential energy, greater complexity of structure and higher refinement of texture. Since the building of atoms into molecules involves the absorption of the energy which does the building, every additional atom in the molecule means additional inherent energy."

In the September, 1909, number of the *Nature Cure Magazine* we wrote as follows:

"It is vital force manifesting through the life elements in the plant, animal or man which, in conjunction with the light, warmth and energy supplied by the sun, elaborates the elements of the earth and air into the ascending forms of life and consciousness. In other words, vital force or the life element is the builder, while sun heat and light are building materials."

These processes of metabolism — of building up and tearing down — the transformation of one form of life into another — are well described in the following paragraphs translated from a German book on vegetarianism. These descriptions reveal the wonderful commerce and reciprocity between the higher and lower planes of life by which the waste products of one kingdom consitute the sustenance of the other. There is no death — life is growth and growth is change.

"This transformation of sunlight into chemical energy takes place in those vegetable cells which contain chlorophyll. (Chlorophyll is a proximate element that gives the green colour to fruits and vegetables). What we call protein, starches and fats are merely different forms of sun energy transformed into chemical energy, and these foodstuffs contain nothing more than sun energy when we consume them in flesh foods. What happens in the vegetable cell? Out of the air, the plant absorbs carbon dioxide. This is a combination of one part carbon and two parts oxygen. To part these elements requires a great expenditure of energy and this work of separation is performed by light or sun energy. The oxygen, which has been torn away from the carbon, escapes into the air and serves as food for the animal and human kingdoms, while the carbon in the plant enters into combination with other elements absorbed from the earth and from the air. Oxidation or combustion is nothing else than the reunion of carbon in the plant molecule with the oxygen of the air. The result is carbon dioxide, which again serves as food for plants.

Sun energy also causes the separation of water into hydrogen and oxygen, and this also involves a great expenditure of energy, part of which becomes latent in the newly formed molecules of the vegetable cell. When in the digestive processes, carbon and oxygen, which have been parted in the formation of the vegetable molecule, again unite, energy is liberated. This storage of energy during the building up processes (anabolism) resembles the accumulation of energy in the wound spring and its liberation while unwinding. On the other hand, accumulation of sun energy takes place in the plant through the combination of carbon with nitrogen and hydrogen. These elements strongly oppose union, but sun energy binds them together. This opposition between nitrogen and carbon is so great that artificially it can be overcome only in the highest known temperatures created in the electric light arc." (Just as it takes a great deal of heat to weld together two pieces of steel.)

From these facts in nature the German author draws the following conclusions which are shared by scientists who defend the materialistic and mechanistic philosophy of life and also by extreme vegetarians who advocate a strictly raw food diet, even to the exclusion of the dairy products. They justify this on the ground that all vital energy in the animal and human kingdoms are derived from sun energy stored in the products of the vegetable kingdom, that human beings, by eating animal food, therefore consume vital energy in second hand and deteriorated form, to which no measureable additions of vital energy are added in the animal and human kingdoms. The author further states these conclusions:

"Thus we see how streams of energy, which the sun sends to our earth, are transmuted into chemical energy; then food is sun energy, and living beings are indeed children of the sun. In the vegetable kingdom only, the springs are wound which drive the mechanism of life. Vegetarians derive their energy direct from nature, while meat eaters obtain energy indirectly in a weakened form. Having studied the transmutation of sun energy into vegetable substance, we understand the meaning of the sentence. "Therefore, in plants we eat sun energy". Without hesitancy we may add to this that in flesh food also we eat sun energy, for the animal builds itself from vegetable food without measurable additions of new forms of energy."

This reasoning may seem plausible from the mechanistic point of view, and has served well the advocates of a strictly vegetarian diet, but unfortunately for the learned author, and for his ultra-vegetarian friends, his arguments are based on false premises and therefore are untenable. The fallacy of his reasoning is due to the fact that the energies at work in the vegetable kingdom are not by any means the highest expression of life force on this planet. On the contrary, the vital energies animating our planetary system, as already explained, manifest in four ascending ranges of vibratory activity. This explains why there is a quality of energy in animal food which cannot be derived from vegetable food, and this something is the animal life principle, animal magnetism, or spiritual life element; in other words, a higher and more refined range of vibratory activity than that which animates the lower kingdoms. The more powerful the vital energy which builds, the more potent the latent dynamic or potential force of the product. Coal, though classed among the minerals, possesses infinitely greater heat and energy producing qualities than other minerals because originally its materials were elaborated under the vibratory influence of the vegetable life element, or vitamin. The latter element ranges much higher in the scale of vibratory activities than the electro-magnetic life element which controls and elaborates the simple compounds and crystals of the mineral kingdom. The animal cell, being synthetized under the operation of the animal life element, is alive with still higher potencies of vital force than those in the vegetable cell. The ascending life elements, or progressive manifestations of vital force, resemble the power of steam at different degrees of tension. Steam at eighty pounds pressure performs work which it could not accomplish at twenty pounds pressure. In similar manner each higher expression of vital force exhibits energies more powerful, and products of greater refinement and complexity than the lower one. The higher the tension of steam, the greater its capacity to perform work. The higher the vibratory tension of the life element, the more potent, complex and refined its manifestations and products. In every higher kingdom of nature molecules become more complex, more refined and possessed of greater potential energy, because the building of atoms into molecules involves the absorption of the energy which does the building. This is illustrated in the formation of ice. The cold which solidifies the molecules of water is absorbed by and becomes latent in the icy crystals which it builds. When the particles of ice disintegrate under the influence of heat, cold is liberated. In similar manner the heat which gives warmth and comfort to our homes is sun warmth which was absorbed in the formation of vegetable cells in the growing plants and trees of primeaval forests, or in the carboniferous matter of annular canopies.

Though these are the facts, it does not follow that we advocate a meat diet. We resort to flesh foods only as a temporary expedient in cases of extreme physical and mental negativity, in order to build up the positive animal qualities which had become greatly depleted. But, for reasons brought forth in this chapter, we do advocate a liberal use of the dairy products in the daily dietary. In these food products of the live animal we partake of the kinetic energy of the animal life element without consuming the poisonous waste matter of the animal carcass. What we commonly call animal magnetism is the animal life element which permeates and animates the animal kingdom. This subtle and potent force, which is not yet present in the products of the vegetable kingdom, is contained in the purest and most available form, unimpaired by cooking, in the dairy products, in eggs and in honey.

While we have discussed the functions of the life elements or vitamins, little has been said about their origin and true nature. In the following chapter we shall endeavour to throw some light on this aspect of the problem.

CHAPTER XI

WHAT ARE THE LIFE ELEMENTS?

There are two prevalent but widely differing conceptions of the nature of *Life* or *Vital Force* – the material or mechanistic, and the vital. The material conception looks upon life or vital force with all its physical, mental and psychical phenomena as manifestations of the electromagnetic and chemical activities of the physical-material elements composing living organisms. From this point of view, life is a sort of spontaneous combustion, or as one scientist has expressed it, a "Succession of fermentations". A well known physician in one of his lectures recently made the following statement: "Every life expression, be it physical, mental, moral, or the so-called spiritual, is a result of chemical action. Even the life force or vital energy has its origin in chemical activities and nothing else." According to this conception the brain oozes thoughts and feelings like the liver secretes bile or the stomach digestive ferments. However, this materialistic conception of life has already become obsolete among the more advanced biologists as a result of the wonderful discoveries of modern science, which are fast bridging the chasm between the material and the spiritual realms of being. But medical science, as taught in the regular schools, is still dominated by the old, crude, mechanical conception of vital force; and this, as we shall see, accounts for some of its gravest errors of theory and practice.

The vital conception regards life as the primary force of all forces coming from the great central Source of all intelligence and creative power. This force, which permeates, heats and animates the entire created universe, is the expression of the "divine will", the "Logos", the "word" of the Great Creative Intelligence. Our sun is one of the millions of power stations for the distribution of this divine energy which sets in motion the whirls in the ether, the electric corpuscles and ions that make up the different atoms and elements of matter. These corpuscles and ions of which the atoms are composed are positive and negative particles of electricity. Electricity is a form of energy. It is intelligent energy; otherwise it could not move with that same wonderful precision in the electrons of the atoms as in the suns and planets of the sidereal universe. This intelligent energy can have but one source — the one and only Source of all life, intelligence and creative will in this universe. If this Supreme Intelligence should withdraw its energy, then the electrons and ions (electrical charges), and with them the atoms and elements — the entire universe would disappear in the flash of a moment.

From this it appears that crude matter, instead of being the source of life and of all its complicated mental and psychical phenomena (which assumption, on the face of it, is absurd), is but an expression of the Life Force, itself a manifestation of the Great Creative Intelligence which some call God, others Nature, the Oversoul, Brahma, Prana, the Great Spirit, and so forth, each according to his best understanding. It is this Supreme Intelligence and power, acting in and through every atom, molecule and cell in the human body, which is the true healer, the *vis medicatrix naturae*, which always endeavours to repair, to heal, and to

51

restore the perfect type. All that the physician can do is to remove obstructions and establish normal conditions within and around the patient, so that the healer within can do his work to the best advantage.

This life force is the primary source of all energy — that from which all other kinds and forms of energy are derived. It is as independent of the body and of food and drink as the electric current is independent of the glass bulb and the carbon thread through which it manifests as heat and light. The breaking of the incandescent bulb, though it extinguishes the light, does not in any way diminish the amount of electricity back of it. In a similar manner if the physical body "falls dead", as we call it, the vital energy keeps on acting with undiminished force through the spiritual-material body, which is an exact duplicate of the physical body, but whose material atoms and molecules are infinitely more refined, and vibrate at infinitely greater velocities than those of the physical-material body. This is not merely a matter of faith or of speculative reasoning, but a demonstrated fact of natural science. When Saint Paul said (1 Corinthians 15:44): "There is a natural (physical) body, and there is a spiritual body", he stated an actual fact in nature. Indeed, it would be impossible to conceive of the survival of the individuality after death without a material body to serve as the vehicle for consciousness, memory and the reasoning faculties, and as an instrument for physical functions. Therefore if survival of the individuality after death be a fact in nature, and the achievement of immortality be a possibility, a spiritual-material body is a necessity.

Sir Oliver Lodge says that the substance of the spiritual body is ether. This is unthinkable. The ether is impalpable and omnipresent. It is, as far as science now knows, the primordial universal element which permeates and enters into the composition of all matter. But ether alone cannot and does not constitute matter. The atoms of the various elements are made up of negative electrical charges, or electrons, vibrating around positive centres, tearing with them the ether like the force of the eddy tears along with it the water. This is true of spiritual matter as well as of physical matter. The only difference between the two is that the atoms and molecules of spiritual matter are infinitely more refined and vibrate at higher velocities than the atoms of physical matter. The sensory organs of the spiritual body are attuned to these higher and finer vibrations. From the foregoing we learn that modern science verifies the wisdom of Pythagoras, who taught twenty-five hundred years ago that all matter was made up of three elements — substance, motion and numbers. According to modern science, the "substance" of Pythagoras corresponds to the universal ether, "motion" to electricity, and "numbers" to the number of electrons vibrating in the atom and to the number of atoms in the molecule.

Those who deny the existence of matter and of material bodies are also mistaken. Matter is as necessary to Being as soul. Soul, the individual spark of cosmic, creative intelligence — the entelechy of Plato, the "thing in itself" of Kant — cannot manifest in palpable, visible form, except in and through matter. Matter forms the material clothing of physical, astral, spiritual and celestial bodies, and these are instruments for the manifestation of life and its vital phenomena. Matter is just as real in the astral, spiritual, celestial and inter-planetary worlds as on this earth plane. As a matter of fact, we are here and now in the spiritual world as much as we ever will be, though matter on this plane is coarser and slower in vibration than in higher spheres of spiritual life. Without its clothing of physical or spiritual-material bodies, soul could not manifest to other souls nor produce or experience an infinitude of material activities and phenomena. Universal or Cosmic Intelligence, the great father soul of all souls, creates individual centres of creative intelligence by incarnating in mineral, vegetable, animal and human bodies. Thus the word, or Fiat, of Creative Intelligence takes on the flesh of matter.

CHAPTER XII

RELATIONSHIP OF MINERAL SALTS TO VITAMINS

Some years ago we stated that the mineral salts were the carriers and conductors of the electro-magnetic energies in vegetable, animal and human bodies, while the negative elements of starches, sugars, fats and proteins were poor conductors. We predicted that one of the next important discoveries of orthodox science would be that the mineral elements are carriers and conductors of vitamins. This prediction seems to be confirmed now by the researches of Dr. Funk and other investigators of vitamins. These scientists claim that they have separated the vitamins and that they appear in the form of tiny crystals. Since minerals assume the crystalline form, it must be mineral elements which bind and conduct the electro-magnetic (and vitochemical) energies in living bodies. This theory is further confirmed by the fact that the mineral elements, as well as the vitamins, are found in greatest abundance in the dark layers and coverings of cereals and rice and in the rinds of fruits and vegetables. This further justifies the preference of the advocates of natural diet for whole grain products, while the medical profession has always ridiculed the idea and claimed that whole grain bread was unwholesome, too coarse for the digestive organs and not fit to eat. Woods-Hutchinson, one of the orthodox "authorities" on dietetics, in his popular articles in newspapers and magazines has for many years denounced whole grain bread as "poison bread". During the late war, while the government forced the stay-at-home public to live on all sorts of combinations of more or less whole grain cereal foods, the soldiers in the camps and trenches, who needed the vitamins even more than did the civilians, were fed on white flour products.

It is interesting to note that the discoverers of the vitamins have verified practically all the claims of Natural Dietetics as to the superior value of raw food over cooked food. Casimir Funk and others report that experiments with various foods on animals languishing and dying from lack of mineral salts and vitamins have shown the following results: (1) Fresh vegetables exhibit greater vitamin activity than any other class of food. It is lowered by cooking and partly lost by drying. Dried dandelions were found to be inactive, while dried cabbage retained considerable vitamin activity. Lemon, orange and other citrus fruits retain the life element even when cooked. This confirms the high estimate we have placed on fruits and vegetables as purifying, antiseptic, tonic and blood building foods. (2) Milk is highly charged with vitamins but cooking destroys them. Even pasteurization or sterilization diminishes them considerably. Condensed milk has lost vitamin A entirely and retains only small amounts of B and C. Cow's milk contains more of the life elements in summer than in winter, and more when the animals are kept on good pasture than when fed on fodder. (3) Potatoes, carrots and other roots are rich in vitamins B and C and partially retain them after cooking. This is the reason why scurvy, which at one time was almost universal in European countries, disappeared after the introduction of potatoes from America. The best and quickets cure for rickets consists in a diet of fresh fruits and leafy vegetables and nuts. (4) In cereals the mineral salts and vitamins are contained chiefly in the pericarps and germs. Thus orthodox science confirms, one after another, the claims and teachings of Nature Cure philosophy and practice, which formerly were either ignored or denounced as vapourings of ignorant tyros and fanatics.

Ever since we began to lecture and write on Natural Dietetics we claimed that the leafy juicy vegetables were richer in mineral elements, and therefore also in life elements, than fruits; that the germ and pericarp of cereals contained the mineral elements and life elements; that potatoes were more wholesome than cereals because they contained considerably less starch and protein and much more mineral matter than the latter; that the boiling, and even pasteurization, of milk kills more or less completely the life elements in milk and thus lowers its nutritive properties. Alfred McCann in his recent work, *The Famishing World*, makes the following statements: "Prior to 1912 (that is before the publication of his first book) the only thing the public ever heard of in connection with a description of food was the academic division made by dieticians. This division consisted of three groups — carbohydrates, proteins and fats. There was another division to which some of them, on rare occasions, slurringly referred. They called this fourth division 'ash'. The division 'ash' was always exasperatingly ignored and apparently had little if any meaning for dieticians and was not considered by them as significant or important." While we can have no desire to detract from the great service which McCann has rendered by spreading the knowledge of a new and better system of dietetics it must be pointed out that most of the information which he gives and the ideas which he expresses are not as new or original as he seems to imply. As early as 1907 these ideas had begun to be publicized in the Nature Cure Magazine and in such books as *The Folly of Meat Eating* by Otto Carqué. Also Julius Hensel, Schuessler, Dr. Lahman and many other pioneers of the Nature Cure movement had taught, as long as forty years ago, practically all that McCann presents in his books, though they were not aware of the existence of life elements or vitamins, of microzymes and their enzymes and ferments as described in the books of our Library of Natural Therapeutics.

Microzymes and Their Relationship to the Vito-Chemical Life Element

There is still another aspect to the vitamin problem which is not generally known. In Volume I of the *Natural Therapeutic* series we have outlined Professor Béchamp's discoveries, according to which the cell is not the smallest single unit of life. This great scientist taught that the cell is made up of minute living beings — microzymes, or minute ferment bodies. According to his theory, the microzymes are the primary units of life. The chromatin or chromosome of the cells and the fibrin of the blood consist of these infinitesimally minute living bodies, and their secretions are the enzymes and ferments on which depend the multitudinous processes of metabolism in living matter. The vito-chemical life element manifests in and works through these primal architects of life and their vital secretions. The microzymes in the cells and tissues of raw vegetables or raw animal foods secrete the enzymes or ferments which help to make possible the digestion of these foods; but the microzymes and their digestive ferments are killed by overheating, boiling or roasting. Thus the food is made less digestible by cooking and the work of the digestive organs is greatly increased thereby.

Raw Food Diet, Pro and Con

The difference between raw and cooked foods is the same as that between live and dead bodies. A cooked apple planted in ever so nutritious soil will not give birth to an apple tree. Its life and sex elements have been destroyed by overheating; thus also some of its finest food values have been dissipated. Raw food contains its own digestive ferments, while in the cooked food these have been killed in proportion to the more or less prolonged exposure to excessive heat. The "discoverers" of vitamins tell us that minute quantities, almost homoeopathic doses, of these life elements are sufficient to cure animals languishing in the last stages of beriberi and similar diseases, and that acid and subacid fruits and leafy, juicy vegetables are richer than any other foods in these life sustaining substances. This explains why it is not necessary to exclude cooked foods from the diet altogether. The vitamins and microzymes of raw foods will assist in the digestion and assimilation of a considerable amount of cooked food. In other words, it is sufficient if a fair proportion, say one half, of a meal consists of raw food and the other half of cooked food. However, these revelations concerning vitamins and microzymes make it clear that, on the whole, the nearer we come to raw food diet, the better it will be for the creation and maintenance of physical and mental health and vigour.

The knowledge so far gained about the true nature of the life elements or vitamins will enable us to expose another fallacy of orthodox food chemistry and dietetics, namely, the fallacy of the calorie.

CHAPTER XIII

THE FALLACY OF THE CALORIE

In the domain of orthodox food chemistry and dietetics the calorie reigns supreme. In colleges, hospitals and sanatoriums practically the only criterion of food values is the calorie. The inflated reputation of this problematical individual rests on the assumption that all animal heat and energy is derived from the combustion of certain food materials. Hoover, the official in charge of the government food administration during the First World War, and his assistants were completely under the domination of the calorie. In their estimates of food values they considered only the heat producing capacity of foods; the all important mineral elements and vitamins they ignored entirely. In the largest sanatoriums in this country, and in many restaurants where the ambition is to be up-to-date in matters of food valuation, the menus indicate in calories the heat producing capacities of the various foods. The accompanying instructions run somewhat as follows: "Your body produces daily a certain amount of animal heat and working energy, and this must be supplied by the food you eat and drink. Your physician will tell you how many food calories or heat producing food units you need per day. Select and combine your foods according to their calorie values in such a way as to provide the necessary fuel materials." The mineral elements are not even mentioned on these menus.

According to the calorie theory, meat, eggs, gluten, starch, fats, oils, cornstarch, glucose and white sugar rank highest as heat producing foodstuffs, while fruits, berries, leafy vegetables and hulls of grains are so much waste, good only for creating acidosis, indigestion and flatulence, and for increasing the already extravagantly high cost of living. Since this may sound like exaggeration, we will say that we had occasion lately to examine the diet prescribed for two diabetic cases, given by physicians in one of the largest sanatoriums in this country. They read as follows: "Meat permissable once or twice a day, eggs also; forty percent gluten bread and butter; no acid or subacid fruits; vegetables must be boiled and strained twice or three times before serving." Such a diet has one certain result — it kills the patient. Diabetes is caused or aggravated by excessive acidity, and all the foods in this prescription are made up of nothing but acid producing elements. The soldiers and sailors of the German raider Crown Prince Wilhelm, which surrendered in 1917 to the United States authorities in Norfolk harbour, had been living for two hundred and fifty-five days on the richest of high calorie foods, with the result that the crew became disabled and the commander was compelled to surrender to a neutral power. When the cruiser steamed into Norfolk harbour many of the crew had found watery graves, one hundred and six were ill in their bunks and another large number were on the verge of breakdown. The ailment from which they suffered was similar to beriberi or pellagra. Prominent symptoms were emaciation, loss of strength, neuritic pains, dropsical swellings and nervous breakdown. When, following the suggestions of Alfred McCann, these men were fed on fluid extracts of bran and potato peelings, on fruits and fresh leafy vegetables, they began to improve immediately and every one of them made rapid and complete recovery. Here is the explanation: the raider, before sinking captured vessels, would relieve them of abundant stores of fresh meats, white flour, potatoes, granulated sugar, salted and smoked meats, condensed milk, breakfast foods, crackers and cookies; but raw cereals such as wheat, maize and barley were sunk with the rest of the cargo. Had the crew taken and eaten the whole grain cereals, and the potatoes with their skins, instead of the meats and devitalised and demineralized white flour products, polished rice and white sugar, they would have remained in good health.

During the last few years hundreds of experiments carried out by scientists all over the world have proved invariably that animals fed on white flour, polished rice, pearled barley, pure starch, proteins, fats or refined sugar develop diseases similar to beriberi, pellagra, scurvy, rachitis, anaemia, decay of teeth and pyorrhoea. The test animals become emaciated, lose strength rapidly and die within two or three months. But they can be cured easily enough, even when near dying. Minute quantities of the polishings of rice, or the bran of cereals, or fresh fruits and vegetables, will revive and restore them to health. In all such experiments the high calorie foods are found to be poison foods, while the despised low calorie fruits and vegetables and the polishings and bran of rice and cereals are the natural remedies and life savers.

The meals served to the crew on the German raider were made up of the following foods: Breakfast: cheese, oatmeal, condensed milk, sausage, fried potatoes, corned beef, smoked ham, fried beef, beef stew, white bread, cookies, butter (oleo), coffee, white sugar. Dinner: pea soup, potato soup, beef soup, lentil soup, roast beef, fried steak, pot roast, salt fish, potatoes, canned vegetables, white bread, soda crackers, cookies, butter (oleo), coffee, condensed milk, white sugar. Supper: cold roast beef, fried steak, corned beef hash, beef stew, potatoes, white bread, sweet cookies, butter (oleo), coffee, condensed milk, white sugar. The average working man would say: "These are the kinds of food that I need; I am working hard and need nourishing food like that to keep up my strength. Fruits and vegetables may be good enough for sick people and idlers, but meat, eggs, potatoes, bread and butter are the foods for me". Yet these rich and nourishing foods came very near killing the entire crew of the raider ship.

Why did not the fresh meat, of which they had an abundance, sustain the crew in good health? In animal bodies the heat producing elements, the proteins and fats, are located in the fleshy tissue, while the mineral elements, the carriers of the vitamins and neutralizers of systemic poisons, are present in the bony structures and in the blood; but these are discarded as waste. To be consistent meat eaters we should, like the carnivourous animals, devour the blood and crunch the bones in order to absorb with the meat a sufficient amount of minerals, Meat carefully drained of blood is excessively rich in protein matter but very deficient in mineral salts. The poisonous waste of the animal carcass are all consumed, while the mineral salts are wasted and the minute quantities of vitamins in flesh foods are effectively killed and dissipated by the boiling, roasting and spicing necessary to overcome the unpleasant taste of raw meat. Ham, bacon, sausage, corned beef and other salted and smoked meats rank high in caloriè value. Why did not these keep the famishing sailors alive? Because they are more lifeless than fresh meat. The salt brine leeches the minerals and vitamins out of the meat and the organic minerals are replaced by the inorganic mineral salt of the brine. It is thoroughly demineralized and devitalized food.

What about the cereal food? The men had plenty of white bread — "the staff of life" — cookies and crackers, all high calorie foods. In cereals the mineral salts and with them the vitamins are located in the pericarps or husks and in the outermost dark layer of the kernel, also in the germ which contains the sex element of the grain and which is charged more than any other part of the kernel with enzymes, ferments and vitamins. As the seed decomposes in the soil under the action of warmth and moisture, the diastase changes the starch into sugar and the peptase changes the protose into peptones and proteose. As the white of the egg and the yolk serve as food for the growing chick, so the sugar and peptones, elaborated by the ferments in the kernel of the grain, decomposing in the soil, serve as food for the rootlets and the young stalk. The refining process in the modern roller mill, in order to produce the "beautiful" snow white flour robs the grain of the hull and germ with their mineral matter, vitamins, enzymes and ferments. These most valuable constituents of the grain are thrown into the bran, shorts and middlings, and the public consume the residue, which will kill chickens, pigeons and other test animals in two or three months' time. Polished rice, pearled barley, and decorticated corn products, deprived of the pericarps and germs, have the same effect as white flour. They are denatured foods, incapable of sustaining life and health.

White or Denatured Sugar: Sugar sap, as it comes from the cane or beet or from the maple tree, is one of the finest and most perfectly balanced of nature's food products. The sugars in these liquids are chemically blended with proteins and the most valuable mineral salts. While passing through the modern refinery the sugar molecules are separated from the proteins and mineral salts. The more nearly the finished product comes to being chemically pure sugar, the more highly it is valued commercially. The sugar itself, however, has been reduced to an inorganic mineral condition, which is revealed by its perfect crystalization. Live colloid substances do not crystallize; they are amorphous (formless). The valuable organic mineral elements, ferments and vitamins found in the sap have been destroyed and eliminated by treatment with heat and chemical poisons; what is left is dead, inorganic matter. The pure sugar molecules, composed of negative elements (COH) only, by the law of chemical attraction leech the mineral elements, particularly iron, sodium, calcium (lime) and potassium from the fleshy tissues and bony structure of the body, thus producing rachitis, scurvy, beriberi, pellagra, anaemia, decay of the teeth, pyorrhoea, and what is commonly known as haemophilia, or a tendency to bleeding. White sugar is infinitely more injurious than white flour. White flour and other denatured cereals are produced by soaking, brushing, pearling, scouring and degerminating, which removes most of the vitamins by mechanical processes, but does not kill the life elements which remain in the finished product. The heat and chemical processes employed in the sugar refinery kill the vitamins and separate the mineral elements, protein and other substances from the sap, leaving nothing but the pure sugar crystals robbed of mineral elements and the life sustaining vitamins. ([1])

During the Civil War, in certain sections of the South which were suffering from great scarcity of foodstuffs, negroes were forced to live for long periods on practically nothing but the juices of the sugar cane. It was found that notwithstanding this one-sided diet, they maintained perfect health and full working capacity. On the other hand, it has been proved that animals fed on refined sugar, white flour or polished rice only, die more quickly than other animals which receive no food at all. It is the general substitution of refined sugar and decorticated corn products for the old-fashioned cane syrup which explains, to a large

---

[1]
  Lindlahr would appear to use the word haemophilia more loosely than is usual in medical literature and to apply it to all forms of abnormal and profuse bleeding. Its use has generally been confined to the hereditary and familial condition in which the tendency to constant and dangerous bleeding has appeared in the males of certain families (notably the Russian royal family) being transmitted through the females who are themselves not affected. Lindlahr would seem to imply that all forms of abnormal bleeding, including prolonged menstruation, dangerous nose bleeds and excessive bleeding from wounds, may generally be traced to the use of devitalized and adulterated foods and should be treated accordingly by a radical reform of diet.

extent, the steady increase in pellagra, rachitis, anaemia and tuberculosis in portions of our population which subsist largely on such demineralized and devitalized foods. The prevalence of haemophilia among women of the wealthier classes of the South is undoubtedly due to similar influences. For generations they have lived on flesh foods, denatured cereals, refined sugar, adulterated candies, ice cream and rich pastries. These devitalized and adulterated foods have robbed their blood of the mineral elements which impart tensile strength and stamina to the fleshy tissues; consequently they have become so weakened that they cannot retain the blood. It streams forth on the slightest provocation, causing profuse and prolonged menstruation, dangerous nose bleeds and excessive haemorrhages from insignificant wounds. Finally it should be noted that honey is one of the finest sugars in nature. It is not generally known that it is animated, not only by the electro-magnetic and vito-chemical life elements, but also by the animal life element which it absorbs from the body of the bee.

Condensed Milk: Milk is nature's perfect standard food. There was plenty of condensed milk in the store rooms of the German raider. Why did it not avert the dread beriberi? The condensing process, conducted at high temperature, most effectually kills most of the vitamins and precipitates the mineral elements, reducing them to inorganic form. The same thing is true of the preparation of the canned vegetables. In the canning process vegetables are subjected to steaming at excessive temperatures. This leeches the minerals, reduces them to inorganic form and kills the vitamins. McCann says in his report that what little the raider captured of fresh fruits and vegetables went mostly to the officers' table. The best part of the food supply was potatoes, but these were robbed of most of their minerals and vitamins by the peeling and boiling. If the sailors had eaten the peelings of the boiled and baked potatoes, or soups made from them, these might have averted the disease in many instances.

Why is it that the long continued agitation of the Nature Cure people has not succeeded in bringing about more extensive production and consumption of whole grain cereal products and of natural unrefined sugars? The reason is that millers and sugar refiners have strenuously and systematically opposed the introduction of more sensible and rational processes. Why should these people uphold the continuances of practices which yearly demand more victims in death, or chronic invalidism than a bloody war? Day by day science traces anaemia, rachitis, tuberculosis, scurvy, beriberi, pellagra, rheumatism and all other chronic diseases more directly to the consumption of denaturalized and devitalized food products. Still, in spite of all protests, the murder of the innocents continues without abatement. Every journal published by millers and sugar refiners ridicules the "crazy ideas" of food reformers, and they use their powerful influence in high places to defeat any legislative measures or government regulations which might interfere with their nefarious practices. Where the saloon killed its hundreds, the roller mill and sugar refinery kill their thousands and hundreds of thousands. The day is fast approaching when these facts will be recognised and the public will be protected against these insidious enemies starving and killing their victims from behind the ambush of commercial greed and expediency, of public indifference, and scientific incompetence and venality.

The question may be asked: "why are the millers and refiners interested in upholding the manufacture of denatured products?" The answer is this: because they would have to scrap their present costly apparatus constructed for the manufacture of devitalised foods, and replace it with new machinery; because their present ways of selling and distributing would have to be revolutionized and superseded by new methods; and, chiefly, because the natural food products containing the native enzymes, ferments and vitamins would not keep indefinitely in the warehouses and on the shelves of the grocery, as do the devitalised white flour, polished rice and white sugar. The vitamins and their live ferments cause fermentation and decomposition, and this increases the risk of deterioration, necessitates quick replacement and increases the cost of handling. This cost, however, would be offset to a considerable extent by simpler and cheaper machinery and manufacturing processes.([2])

The importance of the problem becomes apparent when we consider that the enzymes, ferments and life elements which cause fermentation and decomposition in the whole meal and natural sugar assist in the digestion of these foods in the human body and greatly increase their health and life sustaining qualities, Whole grain meal needs but little yeast to lighten it. Its native diastase and peptase predigest much of the starch and protein constituents, thus facilitating digestion and assimilation. Whole grain meal produced from cereals, rice or legumes, and natural sugar as it comes in fruits, honey and in the sap of the maple, cane or beet, though they are not perfect food combinations in and of themselves, will sustain life and health indefinitely; while denatured and devitalised sugars are not only incapable of sustaining life and health, but actually rob us of these most valuable possessions.

The whole question of the preservation, storage and processing of foods is a very complex one and it has become more so in recent years because of the "advances" which have taken place in food technology. There can be little doubt that the desirable thing is that food should be eaten as far as possible fresh and in its natural state, but this is an ideal which is hard to attain in a complicated and urbanized society and in areas where there are long winter seasons during which food cannot be obtained directly from the ground or from the trees at all times. The classical food preservatives used by our ancestors were salt, sugar and vinegar while sun-drying and smoke curing have also been used for centuries.

These methods still persist to a certain extent but it would probably be true to say that now most of the best preservation of food is done by some form of refrigeration or freezing. Nearly every household now has a refrigerator and many have also a deep freezer. The use of these does not to any great extent reduce the nutritional value of the food, though some fruits and vegetables which do not have a firm structure may be rendered mushy and unpalatable by deep freezing. Commercially various forms of quick freezing and freeze drying are employed and the products thus provided are on the whole good though there is some loss of vitamin content. There is, however, a process known as "blanching" which consists in a short exposure to steam heating at high temperature which is often used as a part of the freeze-drying technique. This leads to a greater loss of vitamins and a destruction of enzymes, though the product tends to keep longer and better. Preservation by drying has a long history. Sun-drying of fruits such as raisins, figs, dates and apricots is extensively used and the smoking of fish and some kinds of meat is common. There are also various methods of artificial dehydration in use which bring about preservation because they check the action of organisms or enzymes which could lead to deterioration. However, most such methods are not to be considered as very desirable especially when sulphuring or "blanching" form part of the process because there can be considerable loss of vitamins and nutrients. Much food, especially fruits and juices, is now preserved by bottling and canning which is done both in the home and commercially. This kind of preservation can produce food which is palatable and of good quality but because it involves heating there is considerable loss of nutritional value, mainly by the destruction of vitamins, though this may not be more than in ordinary cooking. What makes so many canned foods unsatisfactory and dangerous is that they frequently contain chemical preservatives, additives and colouring agents which are harmful to the body and may in some cases even be carcinogenic in tendency. It must be said, however, that some canned and bottled products claim not to have any additives and these should be unobjectionable, though in some cases there may be contamination from the tins. Also, there is a method of preserving developed on the continent which is known as "lacto-fermentation" which by use of a yeast process has an effect on enzymes in the food which leads to the preservation of nutrients and the prolongation of storage possibilities. Irradiation is a method of preservation which is new and which is the subject of discussion and experimentation at the present time. It is likely to be developed and to spread because it has commercial possibilities and could lead to easier and longer storage. It is not, however, regarded with favour by many dieticians as it acts upon the molecular structure of the foods, causes bleaching and destruction of vitamins, may produce so-called "off odours" and may have other dangers not yet revealed.

CHAPTER XIV

VITAMINS OR LIFE ELEMENTS

Names of Vitamins	Diseases resulting from deficiency of Vitamins	Foods containing Vitamins
Fat Soluble A	Keratomalacia Stunted growth of young animals and humans. Rickets or rachitis. Emaciation, weakness, death.	Cream, butter, yolk of egg, cod-liver oil, fat sea-fish, grasses and green leafy vegetables in the order named — spinach, lettuce, tomatoes, cabbage, carrots, sweet potatoes, yellow corn, young peas. In meat only in negligible quantities.
Water Soluble B	Stunted growth, as above. Emaciation, weakness, death. Beriberi, polyneuritis. Pellagra. Rickets or rachitis. Bacteria and parasites. Atrophy of testicles and ovaries. Impotence. Anaemia. Loss of appetite.	Skimmed milk, (not in cream); nuts, green, leafy vegetables; acid and subacid fruits; sweet alkaline fruits; abundant in the germ and pericarp of cereals and legumes; yeast; small quantities in heart, kidneys, liver, brain, negligible in muscular flesh of animals.
Water Soluble C	Rickets, or rachitis. Decay of teeth — pyorrhoea. Scurvy. Bacteria and parasites. Anaemia. Loss of appetite.	Green, leafy vegetables; acid and subacid fruits; in the germ and pericarp of cereals and legumes; alkaline fruits as under vitamin B; and in skimmed milk; not in fat, meat or eggs.

A Summary of Scientific Discoveries Concerning Vitamins

In this chapter we shall describe and explain the results of the latest scientific researches pertaining to the subject of *Vitamins*, and as we proceed the reader may compare these findings of up-to-date scientific research with the teachings of Natural Dietetics as presented in these and former writings. The similarity and, in most instances, identity of conclusions arrived at will be quite apparent. The diagram gives in condensed form the results of vitamin research at this time. Column one gives the names of the three vitamins so far discovered and described; column two, the diseases resulting from deficiencies of these vitamins in the foods of animal and man; column three classifies foods according to their vitamin content. As already explained, the *life elements* of Natural Dietetics are the same as the newly discovered vitamins. When these "impurities" are removed, protein, carbohydrates, fat and sugar, according to allopathic science "the most nourishing of foods" are not only unfit to keep the body in healthy condition but produce emaciation, disease and death.

Orthodox science so far has discovered and described three of these vitamins. (1) Fat Soluble A. (2) Water Soluble B. (3) Water Soluble C.([1])

Fat Soluble A Vitamin

It was discovered in 1912 that no growth could be obtained in young rats when the fat in their diet was derived from lard, olive oil or purified casein but that satisfactory growth did take place when the fat was supplied in the form of fresh butter fat, or egg yolk fat. This "something" which was present in these fats was named Vitamin A (Fat Soluble) and it appears to be very particularly present in the cream of fresh unpasteurized milk and in butter fat. It is very specially associated with growth. The quantity of it in milk depends very much upon the feed of the cow. It increases when the animal is fed on green pastures and decreases in winter when it is fed on hay, roots, tubers, etc. Other foods which are rich in Vitamin A are yolk of egg, cod-liver oil and sea fish. Sea fish living in water saturated with mineral salts of lime, potassium, magnesium, iron, sodium, chloride and so forth are richer in mineral elements and therefore more positive (as to animal magnetism) than fresh water fish. Sea fish, in fact, contain over forty parts per thousand of mineral matter while fresh water fish contain only about eighteen parts per thousand. Although milk and eggs are perhaps the most obvious sources of Vitamin A it can be obtained as well from various

[1]
Lindlahr lived at the beginning of the period when vitamins were being "discovered" and investigated. It is clear, therefore, that this chapter is out of date and incomplete. More recent research has led to the identification of at least two new vitamins, D and E, and also to the elaboration or subdivision of vitamin B. However, as the chapter would seem to be very sound as far as it goes both in its presentation of facts and its general argument and conclusions, it is included with only a few minor alterations.

Vitamin E is the most important vitamin to be identified in more recent times but it would appear that the vitamins do overlap with each other to a certain extent and that the whole subject of vitamins and avitaminosis is in danger of becoming over-elaborate and over-complicated. The fact would seem to be that if we have a sound and well balanced diet consisting of foods grown on well cultivated and well mineralized soil we do not need to worry about minerals and vitamins because we shall obtain them in sufficient quantity and variety. It is doubtful whether we can ultimately obtain health by having bad eating habits and bad agricultural practices and seeking to counter-act them by massive doses of vitamins.

The importance of Vitamin E in the prevention and cure of cardiac and circulatory troubles has been demonstrated beyond all reasonable doubt by the Canadian group of doctors led by Drs. Evan and Wilfrid Shute. Dr. Shute's book "Vitamin E for Ailing and Healthy Hearts" (published in paperback by Pyramid Communications, Inc, 919 Third Avenue, New York 10022) makes very interesting reading and seems to show that there are circumstances in which Vitamin E should be administered in massive doses, at least for a time.

vegetables and cereals (see diagram on page 64). There seems to be a connection between the colour yellow and Vitamin A. It appears in yellow, but not in white, fats, and in the more yellow plants and roots, giving rise to the probability that it originates as a yellow plant pigment.

Vitamin A corresponds to what we have described as *animal magnetism* or *the animal life element* in that it is readily available in the dairy products and in eggs, and we have always emphasized the importance of the dairy products in natural diet. Simon pure vegetarians who exclude even the dairy products and eggs from their dietary, overlook the fact that there is something in animal food which they cannot derive from vegetable food, and this something is the animal life principle – animal magnetism, or, expressing it in other words, a higher and more refined rate or vibratory activity than is inherent in any of the lower kingdoms. A rational vegetarian diet properly combined, consisting of dairy products, the positive vegetables and fruits with just enough of starchy and protein foods to supply the needs of the body for tissue building and fuel material, will be found to be an ideal diet for human beings, fully sufficient to keep them in health and strength in the most trying circumstances.

Deficiency of Fat Soluble A causes a peculiar disease of the eyes quite frequent among the starving children in Central Europe and Russia. The name of this eye disease is xerophthalmia or keratomalacia. Lack of Vitamin A retards or checks entirely the growth of new born and growing animals or humans and is accompanied by rapid emaciation. It is also supposed to be associated with rickets but this is still disputed by some investigators.

The fact that the flesh of wild animals is much richer in organic salts than that of domestic animals is easily explained when we consider that wild animals live on nutritious, uncultivated grasses, rich in mineral salts, while domestic animals are raised and fattened only too often on devitalized and demineralized distillery, brewery and kitchen slops and other devitalized food materials deprived of their mineral elements. This and the fact that many cultivated pastures and fields in course of time become deprived of their mineral constituents explain why cattle and horses crave salt. This craving is often cited by anti-vegetarians as proof that inorganic mineral salt is a natural food for animal and man. When our farmers learn to follow the advice of the great Naturist, Julius Hensel, and fertilize their fields and meadows with pulverized rocks and minerals as well as with nitrogenous waste of animal and human bodies, so that the products of the soil contain a normal amount of mineral constituents, then will animals and men display less craving for inorganic salt. We have also claimed that the mineral salts were the carriers of the vitamins. This explains why it is now found that cod-liver oil and sea fish are exceptionally rich in Fat Soluble A.

In the matter of stability it has been found by many investigators that heating milk or butter fat to the pasteurizing point, about 160 Fahrenheit, destroys vitamin A. Heating to the boiling point has the same effect on cod-liver oil. This confirms our view that pasteurization kills the animal magnetism or animal life element in milk and makes it unfit for baby food. The teachings of Natural Dietetics as to the superiority of raw food over cooked food are also confirmed.[2]

Water Soluble B Vitamin

The all important Water Soluble B is found almost entirely in plant foods. Deficiency of this vitamin in the food of animals and man produces stunted growth, emaciation, weakness and eventually death in new born and growing animals in a similar manner as deficiency of Fat Soluble A.

It has always been our contention that bacteria and parasites are not the causes but rather result of disease conditions, that the microorganisms of disease grow and multiply to the danger point only in a pathogenic (morbid, disease producing) soil and that a body endowed with pure blood and tissues, good vitality, a good mechanical state and with a constructive mental, emotional and moral attitude is practically immune to germ disease. This contention is now supported by the research in connection with vitamins B and C which has shown that deficiency of these vitamins leads to the development of bacterial types of disease in animals in addition to other symptoms and conditions. Beriberi, pellagra and similar diseases are directly traceable to deficiency of Vitamin B. Rickets or rachitis is caused by deficiency of Vitamins B and C. Lack of Vitamin B produces atrophy of testicles and ovaries and thereby sexual impotence in males, amenorrhoea and sterility in females. This has been verified in many cases among the

---

[2]
D. S. Mackinnon, the disciple of Lindlahr, was very much opposed to the use of cod-liver oil to supply vitamins to humans. He claimed that it contained a great deal of toxic material and that various animals used in experiments had been given very small quantities of it over a period and had died as a result. Others have taken the view that cod-liver oil can be used in certain cases but that it should be administered on its own some hours away from any meal. It is probable that it is best to seek vitamins from other sources and to avoid cod-liver and halibut oil. Moreover when vitamins are administered they should be derived from natural sources and not made synthetically in a laboratory on a purely chemical basis. Lindlahr maintained that a proper natural diet would contain all the vitamins necessary, but there may be an argument for the use of vitamin supplements in some cases, at least as a temporary measure.

starving multitudes of Central Europe and Russia in the post-war period. Practically all forms of anaemia including pernicious anaemia are caused by deficiency of Water Solubles B and C.

Occurence of Vitamin B in Foods

Vitamin B is present in skimmed milk but not in cream or butter. One of the B group, Folic acid, is most abundant in green, leafy vegetables, and not so much in fruits. Nuts contain fair amounts. Large amounts are present in the germ and pericarp of cereals and legumes. Investigators claim that the germ is richer in vitamins B and C than is the pericarp or outer tough covering. It is present in good quantities in the tissues of heart, kidneys, liver and brain but less abundant in the muscular flesh of animals commonly used for food.

Water Soluble C Vitamin

Deficiency of this vitamin, as already stated, creates and aggravates rickets or rachitic diseases characterized by softening and decay of the bony structures, all forms of anaemia, decay of teeth and pyorrhoea. Deficiency of vitamins B and C is responsible for scurvy or scorbutus; they are therefore called anti-scorbutic vitamins. For instance it was reported that a number of cases of infantile scurvy occurred in Prague in 1917 and 1918. This was a post-war phenomenon. The "raw" milk was in short supply and of doubtful "rawness", oranges had disappeared from the shops early in the war and other fruits and green vegetables were difficult to obtain.

Water Soluble C is most abundant (in the order named) in green vegetables, acid and subacid fruits, germ and pericarp of cereals, alkaline fruits, and in skimmed milk. Vitamins B and C are not present in fats, meat and eggs, or only in minute quantities, even in the raw state. Experiments on animals have shown that under a diet deficient in vitamins B and C they develop decay of the teeth and a condition similar to pyorrhoea. This confirms our contention that tooth decay and pyorrhoea are caused largely by deficiency of the mineral elements and vitamins in the conventional dietary.

CHAPTER XV

HOW TO CHARGE FOODS WITH MINERAL ELEMENTS AND VITAMINS

It has been found that various samples of the same kind of fruit or vegetable gathered from different localities differ greatly as to amounts of mineral matter they contain. For instance, a sample of potatoes raised in heavy prairie soil which has been cultivated for many years yielded only thirty parts of mineral matter per thousand of dry substance, while the same kind of potato raised on a rocky and sandy hillside yielded seventy parts of mineral matter per thousand. Any two lots of fruits or vegetables outwardly may look much the same, but differ considerably in their mineral content. This variation depends upon the mineral content of the soil in which the fruit, vegetable or cereal is grown. Julius Hensel, one of the pioneers in the Nature Cure movement, was first to call attention to the fact that the products of garden and farm, as well as animal and human bodies, were starving from a deficiency of mineral matter. He pointed out that in European countries for hundreds, in many places for thousands of years, the soil had been robbed of its mineral elements by intense cultivation and that they had never been restored by adequate mineral fertilization; that the ordinary fertilizers — manure, guano, sewage, filth, and so forth — contain enough of the carbonaceous and nitrogenous substances, but only negligible amounts of the mineral and earthy elements. In order to supply these to the soil he recommended the application of finely ground lava, lime and phosphatic rocks.([1])

In European countries where his advice has been followed by progressive, wide-awake agriculturists crops have been doubled and trebled in quantity, and so have the mineral content of the products. In

([1])
What Lindlahr has to say about maintaining the proper mineralization of the soil is of great interest and importance. Even among those who are committed to an organic type of cultivation and farming this is a matter which does not receive enough attention. Compliance with the "law of return" on which the maintenance of fertility depends must involve not only the use of composts and organic manures but also on taking steps to be sure that the soil of cultivated lands does not become permanently deficient in mineral elements. We must in fact seek to follow or imitate what nature does when water and glaciers grind down and wash down rocks and soil and deposit them in the form of silt in river valleys and estuaries. Julius Hensel was apparently the pioneer in the use of ground rocks in cultivation and Lindlahr also used iron filings and wood ash, as he here explains. However, the use of sea-weed in various forms is something which could be done much more than it is with the same end in view. Sea-weed has been traditionally used as a manure in many coastal regions of the world and now the deposits of calcified sea-weed on the Breton coast are being made available on a commercial scale under the name of Maerle. Similar deposits are known to exist in Galway Bay and elsewhere and tend to be constantly maintained by the sea currents.

our institutions for the healing of the sick we begin the treatment of patients by treating the soil of our gardens and farm lands with mineral fertilizers. In connection with our Elmshurst Health Resort we have been cultivating sufficient garden and farm land to furnish our institutions from spring to fall with vegetables grown on highly mineralized soil. For many seasons now we have saturated the land with wood ash, sifted coal ash, finely pulverized lime rock, pulverized phosphatic rock, iron filings and with small quantities of ground rock salt. Wood ash is to the soil what milk is to the human body. It contains all the minerals in the vegetable kingdom in concentrated form and in the right proportions. When any kind of vegetation is burned, all the negative carbonaceous and protein elements are dissipated, while the positive alkaline bases of iron, lime, sodium, potassium, magnesium, manganese, silicon, and also the earthy sulphates and phosphates, remain in the ash. Sifted coal ash is also a good mineral fertilizer, though not as valuable as wood ash. Coal originally was vegetable matter which contained minerals in the live organic form; it is rich in iron, sulphur and silicon. Lime from the quarries, specially pulverized for fertilizing purposes can contain about fifty per cent lime and other valuable minerals. The value of pulverized phosphatic rock as a mineral fertilizer is now generally recognized by agricultural experts. The addition of this fertilizer alone, has, in many cases, doubled and trebled the crops from land that was supposed to be completely exhausted. Iron filings decompose or rust in the soil and enter into chemical combinations suitable for assimilation by plant life. Black loam soil that has had a tendency to acidity can also stand a moderate amount of ground rock salt. Too much of it would burn the tender plant. We have applied to our garden land from two-hundred to three-hundred pounds per acre. The effect of this continued, systematic, mineral fertilizing on the products of our gardens has been little short of marvellous. Every season our vegetable gardens excite the admiration of those who have the pleasure of seeing them. During a period of four years we have grown over forty varieties of vegetables and, when the weather was seasonable, all of them with splendid results as regards quantity and quality. As a rule, in the average garden a few vegetables do well, while others fail to come up to expectations. The abundance and superior quality of vegetables and small fruits grown on mineralized soil must be due to the fact that each variety of plant finds in such soil the mineral substances it requires. It has been found also that soil, in order to be productive, must be rich in vitamins. These are provided by manures and live, vegetable fertilizers in conjunction with mineral and earthy elements.

During the last few years we have been supplanting the putrefying animal manure with live green fertilizer in the form of winter vetch and rye sown on the fields in the fall as soon as the crops are removed. These grasses are very hardy and keep alive during the winter under the snow. In the early spring they grow very rapidly, and some of the growth may be used advantageously as a good milk producing food for the dairy cows. But the bulk of it should be plowed under. It makes the cleanest and richest all-round fertilizer, rich not only in carbonaceous and nitrogenous substances, but also in mineral elements and vitamins, provided the soil has previously been thoroughly mineralized. The roots of the winter vetch are covered with micro-organisms which manufacture nitrogenous compounds highly valuable as plant food.

The vito-chemical life element in vegetables, fruits and grains grown on highly mineralized soil raises the minerals to the vegetable plane of life and elaborates them in the protoplasm of the vegetable cells and tissues into the live organic substances of the vegetable kingdom. The vitalization of earthy and mineral elements depends upon the presence and activity of microzymes, the minute ferment producing bodies of vegetable and animal cells. Colloid matter is not necessarily living matter. Minerals may enter into chemical combination with carbonaceous and albuminous substances, but this does not produce living matter endowed with the vito-chemical life element. The vegetable and animal life elements act only in and through the microzymes, and these are not present in the colloid compounds made by the chemist in the laboratory. Professor Béchamp, the discoverer of the microzymes, has distinctly pointed out the difference between the so-called "organic" compounds produced by the chemist and the living matter of vegetable and animal protoplasm. He taught that what the chemists call "organic" matter consists of various carbon and protein compounds, which may combine with earthy and mineral elements, while "live, organized" substances are those which are alive by virtue of the microzymes which they contain. He says in his book "Le Sang": "The proximate principles, the colloidal matter of the chemist, are naturally unalterable, and do not ferment even when they are left in water at physiological temperature in contact with a limited quantity of ordinary air. On the other hand, natural organic live matters under like conditions, even when absolutely protected from the atmospheric germs, invariably alter and ferment."[2]

[2]
    Lindlahr based many of his ideas on the writings and researches of Antoine Béchamp, the French scientist who was the contemporary of Pasteur but who took a very different view from him on the problems and phenomena of fermentation, bacteriology and biochemistry generally. Béchamp's ideas have been entirely eclipsed by those of Pasteur and his followers, but there can be little doubt that he was a great scientist whose work and experiments are capable of throwing light on many medical problems. It would appear desirable that his works should be studied afresh and re-evaluated.

The distinction made by the great scientist between the organic or colloidal substances of the chemists and the matter which is actually alive is, to us, as interesting and important as the discovery of the microzymes itself. It confirms what we have frequently claimed, that nature's live foods and medicines in vegetable and animal matter cannot be entirely imitated and replaced by substitutes made by the chemist in the laboratory. The organic matter of the chemist is not alive with microzymes whose ferments produce all the greatest changes in the metabolic processes of a living organism. In order to produce live, organized foods and medicines the chemist must have the power to create microzymes. While we admit that colloid compounds when used in the form of medicines are not destructive like mercury, arsenic, and other inorganic elements in crude earthy form, it is also true that the carbohydrate and protein compounds produced by the chemist in the laboratory cannot take the place of nature's live foods and medicines in vegetables and in animal protoplasm. For this reason the Schuessler mineral "tissue foods" or biochemical remedies, never can fill the place of the products of nature's own laboratory — they are not live, organic substances.[3]

The claims of Professor Béchamp are proved by the fact that colloidal or proximate food substances (both identical in nature) cannot sustain life. As related in other parts of this treatise, it has been proved, long ago, by scientists of the Nature Cure school that animals fed on

[3]
As explained in my note to Chapter XXIV of the Philosophy of Natural Therapeutics there seems to be a slight mystery about Lindlahr's attitude to the Schuessler tissue salts. The question would seem to be whether they should be regarded as a diet supplement or as a remedy working on homoeopathic principles; that is to say, do they work by supplying a deficiency or do they act homoeopathically, to normalize or improve the metabolism in a specific manner? The salts are in fact prepared by a potentizing techique the same or similar to that used in homoeopathy with the result that the amount of the salt actually present is practically negligible. If they are in fact homoeopathic remedies rather than supplements the fact that they are "inorganic" in character would not seem to be important. There is, however, a school of Biochemic Therapy which believes in the administration of mineral substances in considerable dosages where there is an indication that the patient is suffering from a deficiency of such substances. These preparations have been put through a process of trituration which results in the making of a very fine powder. According to the believers in this type of therapy this will make up for the deficiency of the particular mineral or minerals which has been diagnosed, and the very fine form in which the preparations are administered makes them easily assimilable and harmless, and it is contended that there is no difference between minerals taken in this way and minerals which are derived from ordinary foods. While there is no doubt that the body can take on mineral substances in this way to a certain extent, Lindlahr contends that this is not a good way of doing so, and he is suspicious of giving any minerals in "inorganic" form with the possible exception of common salt in small quantities. According to him there is a real difference between the organic and inorganic forms of these substances although the difference may not be detectable by ordinary chemical analysis. For instance, to give such things as iron or iodine in inorganic form may produce some effects which appear good for a time but in the long run is capable of doing harm in the same way as most allopathic drugs do. It may be suggested that iridiagnosis provides a way of establishing whether the form in which a certain substance is being given is harmful or not, for if its is harmful and not congenial to the body it will be almost certain to show in the iris. Lindlahr's contention is that the proper way of getting the necessary minerals into the body is via the soil and food grown in it.

chemically pure starch, white sugar, or other so-called organic or proximate food elements die sooner than animals who receive nothing but water. The obvious explanation is that such "organic" compounds do not contain the microzymes whose ferments are necessary to digest the food materials. The use of the word "organic" when applied to simple colloidal matter of the mineral plane is not appropriate, because the word "organic" according to its derivation and up-to-date dictionary definition, means "pertaining to or of the nature of organisms of animals and plants; having or consisting of organs". It is only vegetable and animal matter that is endowed with the organs of life.

The microzymes are the carriers of the vito-chemical and animal life elements, and the life of the microzymes depends upon the presence of alkaline bases, or salts. This is another proposition of vital importance. Professor Béchamp discovered the microzymes in the chalk cliffs of Senn. When he placed some of this carbonaceous lime compound in a fermentable fluid, fermentation started. This was caused by the microzymes in the lime rock, in which they had been buried probably for millions of years. The chalk itself, like the coral reefs, must have been formed by the mineral excretions of minute water animals, of which the microzymes are the living remains. This shows that these primary units of life, the carriers of the vito-chemical life elements, or vitamins, are practically indestructible except by exposure to high temperature and by contact with powerful protoplasmic poisons.

CHAPTER XVI

QUESTIONS AND ANSWERS CONCERNING VITAMINS

Before completing this brief survey of matters of vast importance to the human race, we shall endeavour to answer a few questions that frequently arise incidental to a discussion of these subjects. A question which is sometimes asked is: "Certain advocates of a strictly raw food diet claim that boiling, roasting and baking kill all the vitamins in foods and make cooked foods unfit for consumption. Is this true, and is it best to live on raw food altogether?" If the claims of raw foods extremists were true, the human race, having subsisted for ages almost entirely on cooked food, would long ago have become extinct. Boiling is only a mechanical process of subdivision; it separates the molecules of a substance from one another, but does not dissolve the molecule into its atoms. Therefore the vitamins that bind the atoms in the molecule are not dissipated by boiling. To dissolve molecules into their constituent atoms requires electricity, high degrees of heat far above boiling point, or chemical agents such as digestive ferments produced by microzymes. To illustrate: boiling changes water into steam, but the particles of steam are composed of H_2O molecules. These can be split into hydrogen and oxygen by the action of an electric current. You may boil sugar as long as you please. The substance in solution will still be sugar, but the action of yeast, or of the digestive ferments in the body, splits up the sugar molecule into alcohol and carbon dioxide, and this process of chemical decomposition liberates the vitamins that bind together the atoms in the sugar molecule. It is this liberation of vitamins that produces heat in a fermenting fluid.

Roasting and baking will destroy all the vitamins in those foods which are reduced to charcoal by firing and heating, but it will not kill the life elements entirely in those particles in the interior of the roast which are heated, but not burned to a crisp. Therefore rare meat retains more of the life elements than when thoroughly boiled or baked. Vegetables and fruits should be boiled or steamed only long enough to soften them. Boiling will destroy the vitamins in meats, eggs and milk more thoroughly than in fruits and vegetables.

Is it Necessary to Live on Raw Food Altogether?

It has been proved by Funk and other investigators that even minute amounts of vitamins in raw food are sufficient to ferment or digest large amounts of cooked food or foods poor in vitamins. This answers the question: "Is it best to live on raw food altogether"? It may be theoretically best to avoid cooked food entirely, but it is not necessary to the maintenance of health, because, as stated before, small amounts of raw food are sufficient to aid the digestion of comparatively large amounts of cooked food. Nevertheless, all that has been revealed in this treatise goes to show that the more nearly we confine ourselves to a raw food diet, the better for the prolongation of life and the achievement of perfect health.

A diet consisting of raw fruits and vegetables only, excluding even eggs and dairy products, may agree indefinitely with persons of a vital temperament endowed with robust, positive constitutions, It will have a tendency to refine their coarser appetites and passions and to modify excessive sexuality. But practical experience as a dietician in an extensive institutional practice has taught that a long continued raw food diet has an excessively attenuating and sensitizing effect upon the majority of those who place themselves under our care and treatment, especially upon those who are in a weakened, negative, nervous condition, low in flesh and animal magnetism. They usually lose flesh and develop a strong tendency to nervousness, negative subjective conditions, and abnormal psychism. These negative effects of a long continued raw food diet are intensified by the total exclusion of dairy products, as advocated by many raw food extremists. At any given time, many of our patients are undergoing more or less prolonged fasts and others are on a raw food or dry food diet. But, as before stated, we find that a radical regimen in most cases is beneficial when continued for a limited period only.

Is it true that yeast is unusually rich in nutritious substances and vitamins and is it advisable to eat yeast several times a day?

An extensive advertising campaign extolling the virtues of yeast has boomed the consumption of this product enormously and is giving rise to many enquiries concerning its nutritive value and vitamin properties. For many years this was not so and we stood practically alone among vegetarians in the defence of yeast and of fermented bread. Now the pendulum has swung to the other extreme. Yeast is heralded everywhere as a highly nutritious food, rich in vitamins, and as a wonderful remedy for many ills. As far as food value is concerned, fresh milk, fruits and vegetables are much richer in the mineral salts than yeast and they contain an abundance of vitamins sufficient for all purposes in the vital economy of the body. A dish of spinach or an orange contains more vitamins than a yeast cake and, surely, in more delicious and palatable form. Yeast is fairly rich in protein matter but runs very low in all other food elements including the mineral salts. Being a powerful fungoid ferment, it is rich in Fat Soluble A vitamins, but it contains only negligible quantities of Water Soluble B and C vitamins. Its therapeutic value lies in the fact that it is an active ferment and therefore aids the processes of digestion and the oxidation of waste products in the colon. It is a valuable digestive tonic and laxative in cases of intestinal indigestion, constipation, and the resulting toxaemia. We have given yeast in such cases with good results, but under no circumstances would we advise the continuous use of it. It would tend to create the "yeast habit" and in the end aggravate indigestion and constipation. While yeast may be used as a temporary paliative, permanent beneficial results can be attained only by making the organs of digestion more active and alive by natural diet and treatment. The consumption of yeast has given good results also in cases of skin eruptions and other symptoms of toxaemia caused by intestinal inactivity and the accompanying absorption of systemic poisons. The ordinary dose of yeast, when its use seems indicated, is one-quarter of a cake one half-hour before the noonday and evening meals.

Why is it that in many cases natural diet does not immediately restore good digestion and assimilation?

Another question frequently raised is expressed as follows: "I have been living for some time on natural food combinations, rich in mineral salts and vitamins, but I am still troubled with indigestion, constipation and the resulting toxaemia and malnutrition. If my diet is correct, what is the explanation?" In the majority of such cases the membranous linings and glandular structures of the digestive organs are in a clogged, catarrhal, or more or less atrophic, semi-paralyzed condition, They cannot digest or assimilate even the best of foods. It is only through thorough, systematic treatment by natural methods that those organs can be purified from clogging morbid matter and revived to normal activity. Whatever helps to accomplish this in the way of hydrotherapeutic applications, manipulative treatment, curative gymnastics, right mental attitude, and so forth, is good Nature Cure treatment. In such stubborn chronic cases it frequently requires the application of all natural methods at our command for weeks or months in order to produce the first natural movement of the bowels and to restore the digestive organs to vitality.

CHAPTER XVII

THE MAGNETIC PROPERTIES OF FOOD

What is electricity and magnetism? This question could be answered by saying: "Everything is electricity". One modern scientist never tires of saying: "There is nothing but electrons" — and electrons are negative particles or charges of electricity. A few thousand years ago Pythagoras and many other wise men and mystics of antiquity claimed that "all matter is made up of three elements — substance (the one primordial substance), motion and numbers." Modern science seems to verify the teachings of the ancient wise men. The discovery and study of X-rays, of radium and radio-activity has revealed the fact that the atoms of all different kinds of matter are made up of negative charges or particles of electricity, called electrons or corpuscles, which revolve around one another without ever touching, as the planets in the starry heavens swing round their central suns. These electrical whirls or vortices tear through the ether (primordial substance) as the centripetal force of the eddy tears through the water. Furthermore, it has been found that the number of the particles of negative electricity (electrons) vibrating in the atom determines the physical qualities of the atom or element. In other words whether an atom or element impresses our sensory organs with the physical properties of iron, carbon, hydrogen, oxygen or of any one of the other elements of matter depends upon the number of electrons in the atom and their modes of vibration. It has been found that the number of electrons or corpuscles in the atom determines its atomic weight. Science, in its wonderful achievement, has gone so far as to count, approximately, the number of electrons in the atoms — at least in the lighter ones. The electrons, or negative charges of electricity in the atom, are accompanied by or surround spheres of positive electricity, and the unit of these positive and negative charges of electricity has been named the "ion". Thus we find the teachings of the ancient wise men and mystics verified by the discoveries of modern science. The primordial substance of Pythagoras is the ether, in various stages of refinement. Motion is the oscillation or vibration of the electrons in the atom, and numbers, the number of electrons or corpuscles which make up the atom of matter.

Science assumes that the electro-magnetically negative atom has more negative corpuscles than are necessary to balance its positive electricity, and that the electro-magnetically positive atom has fewer negative corpuscles than are needed to balance its positive sphere of electricity. It is this deficiency or superfluity of negative corpuscles that constitutes positive and negative magnetism or polarity, which causes the desire of the negative atom to equalize its polarity by union with a positive atom. This is the chemical affinity, or valency (combining power) of the atoms or elements of matter. The greater the surplus of negative corpuscles in the atom the greater will be the desire of chemical affinity for atoms having a deficiency of negative electrons — those which are, in other words, surcharged with positive electricity. Therefore, according to the predominance of the positive or negative qualities in a force, matter or entity, we speak of them as positive or negative. We learn from the foregoing that the law of polarity is fundamental in nature. On the activities which it provokes and regulates is built the entire structure of the universe; the cessation of these activities for the fraction of a second would cause the universe to disappear into nothingness in the flash of a moment. This fundamental law of nature has been expressed in these words: "There is a principle in Nature which impels every entity to seek vibratory correspondence (or equilibrium) with another entity of opposite polarity."

The swaying to and fro of positive and negative, the desire to balance incomplete polarity, constitutes the very ebb and flow of life. All through nature, from the most minute to the greatest and most complex, runs this great dividing line between positive and negative. In the mineral kingdom, polarity manifests in the attraction and repulsion of atoms. In the vegetable, animal and human kingdoms polarity becomes more and more identified with sex. Broadly speaking, the male sex represents the dominant, active, aggressive, positive qualities, and the female sex the negative, passive, receptive qualities, Individuals exhibit all shades, grades and mixtures of these general sexual characteristics. Attraction between the sexes depends upon the innate tendency and desire to equalize unbalanced or disturbed polarity. Exaggerated positive or negative conditions create disease on the respective planes of being. Physical disease, as we have explained in other chapters, is always accompanied by the predominance of the electro-magnetically negative elements and forces. Foods, medicines, suggestion and all other kinds of therapeutic treatment, exert on the individual subjected to them a positive or negative influence. It is therefore of the greatest importance that the physician and everyone who wishes to live in harmony with nature's laws should understand this all important question of magnetic polarity.

Polarity of Food and Medicines

Two principal factors determine the positive and negative qualities of foods and medicines. First in importance is the character and unimpaired activity of the life elements inherent in the foods. The second factor lies in their content of positive and negative elements. Aside from the influence of the life elements, the positivity of a certain food or medicine depends upon its richness in the positive, alkaline mineral elements, in the live organic (vitamin) form. The percentages of the positive and negative elements in the principal foods and food classes are shown in the "Table of Food Analysis". A study of this table confirms what we have asserted and constantly reiterated, namely, that the first four groups of our food classification — the starches, sugars, fats and proteins — when chemically pure, are made up entirely of electro-magnetically negative, acid producing elements, and are therefore negative and disease producing in their effects upon the human body; while the fruits, vegetables and other food products of the fifth or mineral group are exceedingly rich in the positive mineral elements and poor in the negative acid forming elements and have, therefore, a positive, health producing effect upon the system.

We will now consider in how far positiveness and normal function of the human body are dependent upon the positive mineral salts in food and drink.

(1) Iron. Iron in the form of Haemoglobin is all important as a carrier of oxygen from the lungs into the tissues of the body. Combustion is impossible without oxygen, and digestion is a slow process of combustion. Without combustion there can be no heat production nor any cremation and elimination of waste products. Furthermore, it has been discovered that iron and other minerals moving rapidly in a salty solution (sodium chloride in the blood) are concerned in the production of electric and magnetic currents. Therefore iron is one of the most important positive energy producing elements in the body.

(2) Sodium: Carbon, oxygen, hydrogen and nitrogen are the four unstable, negative, gaseous elements in the human body. Three of these — carbon, oxygen and hydrogen — make up the various fuel materials, such as fats, oils, starches and sugars. They are to the body what coal is to the furnace; they liberate heat and energy. Similarly to coal, they give off, in the process of combustion, a great deal of carbon dioxide (CO_2), commonly called carbonic acid, and if this poisonous gas is allowed to accumulate it will extinguish the fire in the furnace, or, the life in the body. The elimination of the carbon dioxide depends largely on sodium, which is a positive alkaline mineral element. It does the work in the following manner; Sodium circulates in the body as disodium phosphate ($N^a_2HPO_4$), that is, in molecules which contain one atom of phosphorus to two atoms of sodium. This combination, however, is a loose one. One atom of sodium to one of phosphorus (N^aHPO_4) forms a stable union, the second atom of sodium being a loose addition. As soon as the unstable sodium atom finds a more powerful attraction it leaves the phosphorus and joins the stronger affinity. Such an affinity for sodium is carbon dioxide (CO_2). These two, when they meet in the blood, form sodium carbonate (N^aHCO_3), but this union also is not a true and lasting one; for when the combination reaches the lungs, the gaseous CO_2 and H desert the sodium and pass, through expiration, into the open air. The sodium now reunites with its old friend phosphorus, but on its travels back into the body repeats the same trick when it again meets CO_2. Thus are enacted at the very foundation of this universe, in the world of atoms and molecules, the same attractions, unions, separations, desertions and reunions as those caused by the friendships, loves and hatreds of human beings.

If sodium is lacking in the blood, CO_2 accumulates and gradually asphyxiates the process of combustion on which depends digestion, heat production and reduction of waste. This condition is indicated outwardly by loss of appetite, malnutrition, loss of weight, coldness of hands and feet, blue colour of lips, nails and skin, all the characteristic symptoms of anaemia, and finally of tuberculosis. In other cases, partial oxidation of food materials and waste products, under the influence of carbon dioxide poisoning, causes fatty degeneration, The food materials instead of being transformed into heat and energy become fatty deposits. Just as insufficient draft in the furnace turns partially consumed coal into clinkers, so in the body partial combustion turns starchy foods into fat instead of reducing them to heat and energy. Therefore the excessive consumption of starchy food, lack of exercise and fresh air, causes fatty degeneration, people thus afflicted often complain: "I eat so little, yet everything seems to turn to fat". This is literally true, for the reason just stated. The cure in such cases consists in prompt elimination of the carbon dioxide; better oxidation through increased muscular activity, fresh air and deep breathing; and an increased consumption of sodium in the organic form found in fruits and vegetables. Thus we are presented with the paradoxical fact that carbonic acid poisoning may cause, according to individual constitutional peculiarities, in one person destruction of tissues by pernicious anaemia or tuberculosis, and in another person an excess of fatty deposits. In fact many cases of tuberculosis are preceded by fatty degeneration, The connection between the two is now plain.

(3) Lithium: The element lithium, though present in the body in small quantities only, performs acid binding and eliminating functions similar to those of sodium.

(4) Calcium (Lime): Lime, in connection with silicon, phosphorus and magnesium, makes over fifty per cent of the bony structure of the body and it imparts tensile strength to all the tissues, If this mineral element is lacking in the daily dietary, the deficiency may result in rachitis and scorbutic diseases, scrofula, a tendency to bleeding (haemophilia), osteomalacia, decay of teeth and diseases of the hair, Like other positive alkaline mineral elements, calcium also serves as a neutralizer and eliminator of poisonous acids.

(5) Magnesium: This element performs functions similar to those of sodium and lime. It is a neutralizer and eliminator of destructive acids. It is also concerned in the liberation of electro-magnetic energies.

(6) Potassium ([1]): This positive alkaline mineral element serves also as a neutralizer and eliminator of acids, alkaloids and ptomaines. Furthermore, it is to the muscular tissues what lime is to the bony structures; that is, it forms the solid basis of the fleshy tissues and imparts to them tensile strength.

This brief survey of the positive mineral elements and their functions in the body explains why foods rich in the organic mineral salts exert a positive influence on the human organism and its functions. It is now apparent why an excess of protein and starchy foods in the daily dietary and a corresponding shortage of mineral salts will inevitably clog the system with waste matter and destructive, poisonous acids, alkaloids and ptomaines. ([2]).

The Relationship of Positive Alkaline Salts to Negative Protein Materials

All protein foods are composed of the unstable negative gaseous elements — carbon, oxygen, hydrogen and nitrogen, and the negative

---

([1])   Charles de Coti-Marsh a physician and dietician who died in 1968 was the originator of a system of diet and treatment which, while it has a wide applicability, was designed particularly for the treatment of arthritis. The diet which he advocates is not very different from that which is recommended by Lindlahr and other diet reformers but he does lay a very special emphasis on the importance of potassium and he attributes calcification and deposits in the circulatory system and in the joints very largely to a deficiency of potassium in the soil, in food and in the blood stream, and he claims that even advanced cases of arthritis can be cured by a strict observance of the regimen which he outlines in his books. The main features of his dietetic regime are the avoidance of salt, tea, white flour and refined sugar products and animal fats. He gives much information on the various foods which should be used and on their preparation and he is very much opposed to the use of aluminium cooking vessels. However, in addition to the regulation of diet his system also involves the use of a number of preparations of a herbal and homoeopathic character of which the most important are so-called "K" tablets to provide the body with more potassium, deep seaweed tablets to provide practically all minerals required by the body in the right proportions and so-called "Energy Plus" tablets mainly containing vitamins. At the beginning of treatment it is very important that the body should be detoxified and the bowels encouraged to work well by natural means, and there are so-called "Detox" tablets and Oil of Garlic tablets to assist in this regard. There are also various Diet Supplements, vitamins and homoeopathic remedies which are recommended for use in cases where they seem to be required. The work of de Coti-Marsh is now being carried on by the Arthritic Association which he founded (19 Manning Avenue, Highcliffe, Christchurch, Dorset BH23 4PW) and the literature and preparations required can be obtained by writing to Hursdrex Ltd, 75 Victoria Street, London S.W.1. The names of the books by de Coti-Marsh which are certainly very interesting and worthy of study are "Prescription for Energy", "Diet for Arthritis", "Rheumatism and Arthritis, the Conquest", "Home Treatment for Arthritis" and "The Marvary Meal". It should be added that de Coti-Marsh believed that manipulative treatment had an important part to play in the treatment of arthritis but he seems to have felt that any forceful manipulation of joints should be avoided in the first stage of treatment and postponed until the mobility and general condition of the tissues and joints had been improved by dietary and general treatment.

([2])   Lindlahr does not here discuss specifically Silicon and Manganese but elsewhere he points out their importance in the economy of the body (see Chapter II.)

earthy elements — phosphorus and sulphur. These foods, being rich in acid producing nitrogen, phosphorus and sulphur, form in the processes of digestion and cell metabolism large amounts of destructive acids and other systemic poisons. These acids, if not promptly neutralized by the positive alkaline mineral bases (especially sodium), accumulate in the system and actually destroy the living tissues. To make this clearer — if sodium is lacking in the blood, the destructive acids satisfy their chemical affinity for alkaline elements by leeching them from bones and muscles, thereby causing the weakening and decomposition of these tissues, as we observe it in the decay of the dentine and enamel of the teeth.

This fact is strikingly illustrated in the English "Banting Cure" for the reduction of fat and flesh. This regimen consists mainly of a lean meat diet with the exclusion of fats, starchy foods and sugar. Such a purely protein diet produces large amounts of the acids of nitrogen, phosphorus and sulphur and is deficient in the acid binding alkaline bases, sodium and magnesium as well as in vitamins. The acids, therefore, break down and destroy the fat, and they also destroy the muscular tissues so that reduction of fat and flesh by such means is a destructive, disease producing process. This explains why people undergoing such cures become weak and nervous and develop various forms of uric acid diseases, such as rheumatism, heart diseases and calculi (stones) in kidneys and bladder. We can also understand why people living almost exclusively on "strengthening" meats and eggs grow pallid and thin, while the immigrant peasant girl reared on coarse bread, roots and vegetables and dairy products, is plump and strong. This also explains why she loses her pink and white complexion after a few years of American "high living".

CHAPTER XVIII

CLASSIFICATION OF FOODS ACCORDING TO THEIR MINERAL CONTENTS AND VITAMIN VALUES

Editor's Foreword

In editing this chapter certain difficulties arise in connection with the Analytical Food Chart which forms an important part of it. There are no less than three versions of the Chart, one of which appears here in Lindlahr's book and two others which seem to be revisions and enlargements of the original made by his disciple, Daniel Mackinnon, and included by him in his writings. There is much valuable material in the later versions which are in some respects fuller than the original, but when the three versions are examined together there are certain differences and inconsistencies between them which it is difficult to reconcile. There would seem to be little doubt that all the versions have originated from the same source, but we do not know exactly what this source was though it would seem probable that it may have been a work by a certain Dr. Lahman who is often quoted by Lindlahr and who was a well-known dietician in America at that time.

So, as it is not possible to go back to this original source, it has seemed best to make up some figures which are lacking or doubtful by reference to official tables by McCance and Widdowson on the "Composition of Foods" obtainable from H.M. Stationery Office. This has not, however, produced an entirely satisfactory result because there are obviously differences in the methods used in food analysis now and in Lindlahr's time. In cases in which figures from this more modern source are used they are printed in italics. However, the Chart in the form in which it is printed, while not being entirely reliable and up-to-date in all details, is nevertheless very valuable as giving a good guide to the chemical composition of most common foods. The dietary system which Lindlahr advocates involves the division of foods into five groups and the classification of recipes by a sort of code which roughly indicates the proportions of each group contained in each recipe.

The use of the Chart can make it possible without great difficulty to take any cook book and classify the recipes in it in the same way as Lindlahr classified the recipes in his own Cook Book, some of which are printed in Appendix VI. It is also possible to see at a glance whether a certain food contains elements which a certain person specially requires or too much of elements which may be contra-indicated. Finally, it may be said it is highly desirable that the Chart should be revised and possibly enlarged in the light of the most modern and authoritative food analyses which are now available. Also the Chart seems to point the way to producing analyses which reveal the quality of foods rather than merely analysing specimens taken more or less at random. Lindlahr seems to have shown that there is a difference in the analysis of potatoes grown in soil rich in minerals and potatoes grown in poor or average soil. Doubtless the same sort of differences could be demonstrated in the case of many fruits and vegetables in

Analytical Food Table Chart

Quantitative and qualitative analysis of food products and their classification

Negative elements in the body – acid producing (C.O.H.N.P.S.Si.Cl.)

Fats and Carbohydrates: Fats, oils, starches sugar, Dextrine, Grape sugar. } C. O. H.. } All Negative } Form carbonic-acid in process of digestion.

This gas when it accumulates in the body impedes and extinguishes the processes of oxidation or combustion, on which depend all other vital functions. It causes the characteristic symptoms of the anaemic, viz.: blue colour of face, lips and nails, shortness of breath and retarded metabolism (vital activity) in general.

Nitrogenous food elements.
- Myosin. As predominant in muscular parts of meat.
- Albumen. As predominant in whites of eggs.
- Gluten. As predominant in dark outer parts of grains and rice.

} O H N P S } All Negative

These food elements, in the process of digestion, form carbonic, uric, sulphuric, phosphoric hippuric acids and various poisonous alkaloids, such as Xanthine, Creatine, creatinine and ptomaines, which become, when not rapidly and thoroughly eliminated, the most fruitful source of diseases.

The Dietetics of the regular schools of Medicine and American vegetarianism deal with fats, carbohydrates and nitrogenous foods only – in other words, with six elements only out of the 15 or more found in the human body.

Positive elements in the body – acid-binding and eliminating (K.Na.Ca.Mg.Fe.)

The amounts of organic salts, because they occur in very small amounts only, are given in parts per 1000 of dry substances.

The destructive, poisonous acids which are the waste products of protein, fatty and starch digestion, must be neutralised by the *positive alkaline mineral* elements before they can be properly and easily eliminated from the body; thus carbonic-acid gas is changed into sodium carbonates, uric-acid into urates, etc. If the neutralising positive alkaline bases are lacking in the blood, the acids draw them from bones and muscular tissues, causing rachitic scorbutic and wasting diseases.

The digestion (combustion) of the proteins, fats and carbohydrates depends on a plentiful supply of oxygen, and this depends on a sufficient amount of iron in the blood.

The metallic elements, iron and magnesium, moving in a salty solution (blood), produce electric and magnetic currents.

Lime, magnesium, fluorine and silicon form the solid framework of the bony structures. The chief organic salts in the blood are sodium chloride, sodium carbonate and sodium phosphate.

A comparison of the analysis of milk and blood shows that in milk the percentages of lime and potassium are much larger than in blood, while in the latter the percentages of sodium and iron are much greater than in milk. The reason for this is that the fully developed organism needs less of the building materials than the new born and growing body, but much more of the eliminating oxygen-carrying and electricity-producing sodium and iron. For these reasons milk is the correct standard for the growing body, while blood is the better standard for the fully developed body

	II	III	IV		V				VI					VII	VIII	IX
	Water	Nitrogenous food elements O H N P S	Carbohydrates COH		Negative, gaseous or mineral elements				Positive mineral elements, acid-binding and eliminating					Totals per 100 of the negative elements in protein and carbohydrate foods in Col III and IV	Totals per 1000 of the positive mineral elements in Col VI	Calories, Heat producing units per pound
Foods	Parts per 100	Parts per 100	Fats Oils	Sugars Starches Dextrines	P	S	Si	Cl	K	Na	Ca	Mg	Fe			
			Parts per 100		Parts per 1000				Parts per 1000							
Human Milk	87.02	2.36	3.94	6.26	7.84	0.33	0.07	6.38	11.73	3.66	6.80	0.75	0.75	12.56	23.69	320
Cow's Milk	87.42	3.55	3.70	4.88	15.79	0.17	0.02	8.04	13.70	5.34	12.24	1.69	0.30	12.13	33.27	310
Eggs	73.67	12.50	12.10	0.55	15.72	0.13	0.13	3.72	6.27	9.56	4.56	0.46	0.17	25.15	21.02	670
Ox Blood	80.82	18.12	0.18	0.03	2.31	1.34	0.35	15.14	3.39	19.80	0.48	0.26	4.14	18.33	28.07	10.13
Lean Beef	72.00	72.00	20.00	0.40	17.00	0.64	0.44	1.56	16.52	1.44	1.12	1.28	0.28	25.40	20.64	800
Sea Fish	80.97	17.07	0.34	1.64	32.03			9.60	18.35	12.55	12.80	3.80		19.05	47.50	
Tomatoes	*94.30*	*0.90*	*0.40*	*3.90*	*0.21*	*0.11*		*0.51*	*2.90*	*0.03*	*0.13*	*0.11*	*0.004*	*5.20*	*3.174*	*105*

X — Classification of foods into positive and negative classes according to the nature of the life elements and to the totals of positive and negative elements

Class I
- Animal foods.
- Positive.
- Animal life element.
- Building.
- Acid producing.
- Milk and Blood.
- 'Standard Foods (children and adults).

Savoy Kale	87.09	3.31	0.71	6.02	4.85	19.25	0.85	17.54	28.07	13.37	33.45	3.60	0.13	10.04	84.00	110	Class II	
Cabbage	89.97	1.89	0.20	4.87	28.04	32.01	0.80	15.04	29.05	14.40	24.80	6.60	0.15	6.96	75.00	115		Vegetables.
Spinach	88.47	2.49	0.58	4.44	19.58	13.18	8.60	12.03	21.71	57.42	22.73	12.20	6.40	7.51	120.46	90		Positive.
Cauliflower	90.89	2.48	0.34	4.55	18.42	8.62	3.37	3.10	40.46	5.38	5.10	3.37	0.91	7.37	55.22	160		Vito-chemical life element.
Asparagus	93.75	1.79	0.25	2.63	16.07	5.36	9.50	5.10	20.74	14.77	9.33	3.72	2.94	4.67	51.50	125		
Lettuce	94.33	1.41	0.31	2.19	16.62	6.87	14.64	13.82	67.94	13.55	26.55	11.20	9.40	2.91	128.64	60		
Carrots	87.05	1.92	0.11	7.43	8.83	4.45	1.66	3.18	25.46	14.63	1.80	3.04	0.70	9.46	45.63	225		
Radishes	93.34	1.23	0.15	3.75	12.03	7.18	1.00	10.10	35.33	23.37	15.45	3.42	3.09	5.13	80.66	75		
Cucumbers	95.60	1.02	0.09	2.28	20.20	6.90	8.00	6.60	41.20	10.10	7.30	4.15	1.40	3.37	64.15	65		
Potatoes[1]	75.48	1.95	0.15	20.72	7.48	2.89	0.88	7.55	26.56	1.33	1.15	2.18	0.48	22.82	31.70	305		(1) From poor soil.
Potatoes[2]	75.00	2.08	0.15	21.00	16.00	6.00	2.00		58.06	3.48	3.16	5.20	1.50	22.13	71.40	305		(2) From mineral soil.
Bilberries	78.00		0.78	5.09	*0.09*			*0.05*	*0.65*	*0.01*	*0.10*	*0.02*	*0.007*	5.87	*0.787*	360	Class III	Berries.
Blackberries	86.41	0.53		4.44	*0.24*	*0.09*		*0.22*	*2.10*	*0.04*	*0.63*	*0.30*	*0.009*	4.97	*3.079*	300		Positive.
Gooseberries	85.74	0.47		8.00	5.72	1.71	0.75	0.22	11.22	2.87	3.54	1.70	1.32	8.90	20.65	205		Acid binding.
Strawberries	87.66	0.54	0.45	7.29	7.97	2.05	7.83	1.10	13.72	18.53	9.23		3.73	8.28	45.21	160		Vito-chemical life element.
Oranges	85.04	0.80		4.50	*0.24*	*0.09*		*0.03*	*2.0*	*0.03*	*0.41*	*0.13*	*0.003*	5.30	*2.573*	235	Class IV	
Apples	84.79	0.36		12.34	4.52	2.81	1.42		11.78	8.61	1.35	2.89	0.46	12.70	25.09	305		Juicy fruits.
Plums	84.86	0.40		8.24	6.03	1.21	1.19	0.15	18.28	3.41	4.34	1.36	0.94	8.64	28.33	390		Positive.
Peaches	84.00	0.65	0.90	11.90	2.67	1.00	0.26		9.63	1.50	1.41	0.92	0.18	13.45	13.64	215		Acid-binding eliminating.
Cherries	79.82	0.67		12.00	5.54	1.76	3.11	0.48	17.94	0.76	2.60	1.90	0.69	12.67	23.89	360		Vito-chemical life element.
Dates	37.00	3.10	0.50	56.00	*0.64*	*0.51*		*2.90*	*7.50*	*0.05*	*0.68*	*0.59*	*0.016*	59.60	*8.836*	1175	Class V	
Figs	17.50	1.34	1.28	69.00	0.53	2.77	2.43	1.10	11.63	10.77	7.25	3.78	0.60	71.62	34.03	1305		
Grapes	78.17	0.59		16.32	3.93	1.41	0.70	0.38	14.16	0.35	2.72	1.06	0.10	16.91	18.39	380		Sweet Fruits.
Olives	30.07	5.24	51.90	28.00	0.46	0.36	0.22	0.06	27.02	2.52	2.49	0.06	0.31	85.14	32.40	2600		Medium positive.
Olive Oil			100.00											100.00		4210		Vito-chemical life element.
Bananas	48.60	1.02	0.50	13.40	*0.28*	*0.13*		*0.79*	*3.50*	*0.01*	*0.07*	*0.42*	*0.004*	14.92	*4.004*	650		Acid binding eliminating.
Raisins	13.10	2.50	3.00	67.40	*0.33*	*0.23*		*0.09*	*8.60*	*0.52*	*0.61*	*0.42*	*0.016*	72.90	*10.166*	1280		
Walnuts	4.68	16.37	62.86	7.89	9.31				6.62	0.48	1.83	2.77	0.28	87.12	11.98	1300	Class VI	Nuts.
Coconuts	46.64	5.94	35.93		2.18	0.95	0.09	2.50	8.21	1.57	8.60	1.76		41.42	20.14	1250		Negative.
Almonds	6.00	23.50	33.06	10.90	14.93	0.12			9.24	0.06	2.90	5.83	0.16	67.46	18.19	1480		Vito-chemical life element.
Peanuts	6.9	19.70	30.40	20.60	*3.70*	*3.80*		*0.07*	*6.80*	*0.06*	*0.61*	*1.80*	*0.02*	70.70	*9.29*	1710		Heating, building, acid forming.
Lentils	12.35	25.70	1.89	53.46	12.60			1.61	12.08	4.62	2.18	0.87	0.69	81.05	20.44	1410	Class VII	Legumes.
Beans	14.76	24.27	1.61	49.01	14.86	1.30	0.25	0.69	15.85	0.42	1.91	2.73	0.19	74.89	21.10	1540		Very negative.
Peas	14.99	22.85	1.79	52.36	0.87	1.03	0.27	0.53	13.06	0.30	1.45	2.42	0.24	77.00	17.47	1560		Heating, building. Very acid producing.
Whole Wheat	13.65	12.35	1.75	67.90	10.90	0.09	0.46	0.07	7.20	0.50	0.75	2.80	0.30	82.00	11.55	1655	Class VIII	Grains.
White Flour	13.40	10.40	1.20	69.40	2.80				1.82	0.08	0.43	0.44	0.03	81.00	2.80	1640		Very negative.
Unpolished Rice	13.11	7.85	0.88	76.50	8.60	0.08	0.42	0.02	3.60	0.67	0.57	1.74	0.22	85.23	6.80	1630		Vito-chemical life element. Heating, building.
Polished Rice	12.55	6.94	0.51	77.61	2.15	0.03	0.11	0.01	0.87	0.22	0.13	0.45	0.05	85.06	1.72	1630		Very acid producing.

By comparing Columns VIII and VII it will be found that most of the foods classed as positive rank not only high in positive mineral elements, but also low in the negative protein, fatty and starchy elements, and vice versa.

accordance with the condition of the soil in which they are being grown and the kind of fertilizers used.

Class I
Animal Foods — Positive

Life Elements: Electro-magnetic; vito-chemical; animal or spiritual.

Milk and Red Arterial Blood, the Only Normal (Standard) Food Combinations in Nature

Properties: Flesh building; blood, bone and nerve building; heating, acid binding and eliminating.

Milk and red blood are electro-magnetically positive foods because, in addition to the mineral and vegetable life elements, they are animated by the animal life element; and because, in proportion to the negative elements, they contain large amounts of positive mineral elements.

Cream and butter contain only the fat of the milk and vitamin A. The sugars, proteins and all the mineral salts together with vitamins B and C remain in the skimmed milk.

Cheese contains the proteins and sugars and more or less of the fats. The minerals remain in the whey.

Buttermilk contains the proteins and minerals, no fat. It is deficient in vitamin A, but contains vitamins B and C.

Sumick contains all the elements of the milk, unless some of the cream has been removed.

Eggs

Properties: Heating, flesh building; acid forming.

Eggs contain large amounts of highly organized fats and protein materials and, in proportion to these, run rather low in the positive mineral elements, especially in the important acid binding sodium. They, therefore, tend to produce in the processes of digestion, large amounts of acids, alkaloids, ptomaines and noxious gases. This explains why stuffing with eggs fails to cure consumption. Tuberculosis and other wasting diseases are aggravated rather than improved by un-natural food stuffing and by drug poisoning.

Storage eggs are especially prone to the formation of ptomaine poisons.

Though comparatively low in positive mineral elements, eggs are classed as positive because they are animated by the animal life

86

element of Fat Soluble A vitamin. They should be used sparingly, and always in conjunction with foods belonging to Group V (Mineral Elements).

Flesh Foods

Properties: Heating; flesh building; acid forming.

Comparative analyses of blood and the muscular parts of animals disclose the fact that, while blood is rich in sodium and iron, bloodless meat (boiled or roasted, as it is usually eaten) is very deficient in these elements and therefore negative and acid producing. Potassium, the principal mineral element in meat, serves as a solid basis for the unstable protein materials of which flesh is composed. Meat eaters, in order to be consistent, should, therefore, like carnivorous animals and primitive races, consume the blood as well as the flesh. Since cooked or boiled meat is deficient in the alkaline salts it creates a craving for inorganic mineral table salt which, however, remains a poor substitute for the organic minerals of fruits and vegetables. Salted meats are much lower in nutritive qualities than fresh meats because the salt brine has leeched out much of the organic mineral salts and vitamins.

The low estimate we have placed on flesh foods is fully confirmed by the discoverers and investigators of the amino-acids and vitamins. Not one of these scientists mention flesh food as an adequate source of amino-acids or vitamins.

Fish

The flesh of sea fish living in water saturated with positive mineral elements (iron, lime, sodium, potassium, lithium, magnesium, etc.) is richer in alkaline mineral elements, and, therefore, in vitamins, than that of fresh water fish and the meat of land animals.

This explains the richness of sea fish and of cod-liver oil in vitamins.

Dr. Lahman and others mention the fact that the flesh of wild animals is much richer in organic salts than that of domestic animals, which is easily explained when we consider that wild animals live on nutritious, uncultivated grasses, rich in mineral salts, while domestic animals are raised and fattened only too often on grasses and vegetable products grown on demineralized soil, or still worse, on distillery, brewery or kitchen slops, which contain no mineral elements.

Class II

Leafy, Juicy Vegetables which Grow In and Near the Ground — Positive

Life Elements: Electro-magnetic; vito-chemical.

Properties: Blood, bone and nerve building; acid binding and eliminating; medicinal qualities.

A survey of our analytical table shows that the foods belonging to this group are much richer in the positive mineral salts than are the animal foods. They are all-important for the maintenance of health, because their positive alkaline mineral elements are the most effective neutralizers and eliminators of poisonous acids, alkaloids and ptomaines produced by the ingestion and digestion of animal foods.

The highly nitrogenous meat diet is not nearly so harmful when properly combined with a liberal amount of green vegetables, as is customarily done in European countries. It is the all-meat-potato-white bread- coffee-and-pie American diet which makes for the prevalence of uric acid diseases, indigestion, constipation, appendicitis, cancer and nervous ailments.

The foods belonging to the leafy vegetable group, on account of their great richness in the positive alkaline mineral elements are the real blood, bone and nerve builders, as explained in other chapters. It has been found that the vitamins of fruits and leafy, juicy vegetables survive boiling much better than those of other food substances. Foods belonging to this group are rich in vitamins A, B and C.

Roots and Tubers

Properties: Heating, blood, bone and nerve building; flesh building; acid binding and eliminating.

Carrots and beets are very rich in dextroses and glucoses, which, next to the fruit sugars, are the purest and finest of natural sugars. They are, therefore, valuable fuel materials. Most of the roots and tubers contain moderate amounts of starches and proteins, but run high in the positive alkaline material mineral elements, which makes them good antidotes to the poisonous acids, alkaloids and ptomaines produced by the highly nitrogenous animal, leguminous and cereal foods.

Some of the roots have valuable medicinal qualities, as explained in Appendix III.

Potatoes run low in proteins (about two percent), but fairly high in starches (about twenty to twenty-five percent). Our analytical table shows that they are not nearly so rich in these elements as are the cereals. However, they rank higher than the cereals in the positive mineral elements, especially in lime and potassium. It is probably for this reason that they are so well liked by children, who need a great deal of these tissue building elements.

The skins of potatoes are especially rich in mineral elements and vitamins and have, therefore, fine medicinal properties. They are palatable when the potatoes are well baked or boiled in the jacket. This shows that the prejudice against the potato existing among medical men and the laity is unfounded. Persons suffering from digestive troubles and malassimilation digest and assimilate the savoury tubers much better than they do cereal foods.

Carrots, sweet potatoes and other red or yellow coloured tubers are rich in vitamin A. All foods belonging to this group have an abundance of vitamins B and C.

Since we wrote the preceding paragraphs many years ago for the *Nature Cure Magazine*, the work of Dr. Hindhede of Copenhagen has fully justified our good opinion of the potato. Dr. Hindhede for many years had been writing about natural dietetics and applying its principles in his practice in accordance with the teachings of the school of Nature Cure.

The reasonableness of his teachings and the practical results of his work were so evident and impressive that during the great food shortage, caused by the late world-war (1914–1918), the Danish government gave him full control over the food situation in Denmark, and made him the national dietitian for the army as well as for the people at large.

He enforced a low protein diet in which potatoes (2 percent protein) largely replaced meat (20 percent protein) and cereals (10 percent protein). The results were surprising. Under the natural food regimen public health improved in a marked degree, and the death rate was lowered considerably. The doctor strongly recommends a more liberal use of potatoes instead of cereals, claiming that this alone is sufficient to cure many diseases.

Class III

Berries — Positive

Life Elements: Electro-magnetic; vito-chemical.

Properties: Heating (according to their content in sugar); blood, bone and nerve building; acid binding and eliminating; medicinal qualities.

Berries, in general, run very high in the positive mineral elements and very low in the negative starches and proteids; they are therefore classed as positive. Some of them, such as the blackberries, raspberries, strawberries, blueberries and bilberries, are rich in highly organized fruit sugars. Their juices contain valuable medicinal elements. They are highly animated by the vito-chemical life element. Bilberries, dried or home canned, without sugar, have great medicinal value in ailments of the intestinal tract. Strawberries are splendid purifiers. When they produce skin eruptions it shows how badly they are needed as eliminators of systemic poisons and scrofulous taints. Persons so affected should live on strawberries until the eruptions cease to appear. They might well follow the example of the wealthy Englishman who liked strawberries so well that he spent his time travelling around the globe following the new strawberry crops from one locality to another.

Class IV
Acid and Subacid Fruits — Positive
Life Elements: Electro-magnetic; vito-chemical.

Properties: Heating (according to their content in sugars); blood, bone and nerve building; acid binding and eliminating, medicinal qualities.

To this group belong all the hardy acid and subacid fruits, such as limes, lemons, pineapples, oranges, grapefruit, tangerines, peaches, apples, plums, pears and cherries. The foods of this group are animated by the vito-chemical life element. They run from medium high to high in the positive mineral elements and very low in the negative starches, fats and proteins. They also exert a positive influence on the organism because they are natural laxatives, cholagogues, purifiers and anti-septics. Their natural sugars are the most easily combustible of all heat and energy producing foods. They are, therefore, the finest natural tonics and stimulants. Distilled in nature's own laboratory, their juices are absolutely pure and the most delicious drinks for man — they are indeed the nectar of the gods. Fruits belonging to this group are exceedingly rich in vitamins B and C.

Class V
Sweet Alkaline Fruits — Medium Positive
Life Elements: Electro-magnetic; vito-chemical

Properties: Heating (according to their content of sugars); blood, bone and nerve building; acid binding and eliminating; medicinal qualities; rich in vitamins.

To this group belong the melon family, cucumbers, grapes and bananas. The foods of this group rank fairly high in the positive alkaline mineral elements and very low in the negative starches and proteids, but they contain large amounts of fruit sugars which are magnetically negative. Therefore we rank them as medium positive. The juices of these fruits have high medicinal qualities. They are splendid natural laxatives and purifiers. Their highly organzied sugars are the richest of fuel materials and natural stimulants and tonics.

Bananas, when well ripened, are wholesome food for children as well as for adults. They run low in protein (one percent) and contain about fourteen percent of starches and sugars. These are well balanced by positive mineral elements.

Figs, dates and persimmons also may be placed in this class, as they are similar in their electro-magnetic and medicinal qualities, to the foods of this group. Figs and dates contain close to sixty percent of fruit sugars which are predigested foods and, therefore, most valuable for those suffering from indigestion, malassimilation and wasting diseases.

Grapes and raisins contain between twenty-five and thirty percent of sugar, with very little starch and protein.

All the members of the melon family are splendid purifiers and contain large amounts of vitamins B and C, though they are not as rich in these as the acid and subacid fruits of Class IV.

Class VI

Nuts — Negative

Life Elements: Electro-Magnetic; vito-chemical

Properties: Heating; flesh building; acid forming.

A glance at our analytical table tells us why these foods are negative. They are exceedingly rich in proteins, fats and carbohydrates, but rank very low in positive organic salts. This explains why nuts "crave salt"; why so many people find nuts "indigestible"; why "fruit and nut" extremists run, physically and mentally, into negative conditions.

Nuts and olives are the natural substitute for meat. They should be used in moderate amounts only and always in combination with foods of the mineral salt group. Olives contain over fifty percent of fat and over twenty-five percent of sugar. They rank fairly high in mineral constituents and are, therefore, more nourishing and wholesome than any flesh food.

The foods of this group contain appreciable amounts of vitamin B.

Class VII

Legumes — Negative

Life Elements: Electro-Magnetic; vito-chemical. The chemicals are located in the pericarp and in the germ.

Properties: Heating; flesh building; acid forming.

Our tables show that the foods of this group run very low in positive mineral elements, while they are exceedingly rich in the negative, starchy and protein elements. In other words, they are very rich in the acid producing starches and proteins and very poor in the acid binding and eliminating alkaline mineral elements. Therefore, if not properly combined with adequate amounts of juicy fruits and green vegetables, they may become as dangerous to health as meats.

The foods belonging to this group contain only moderate amounts of vitamin B and C.

Class VIII

Grains — Negative

Life Elements: Electro-Magnetic; vito-chemical

Properties: Heating; flesh building; acid forming. The vitamins are located in the outer dark layer, in pericarp, and in the germ.

All grains are exceedingly negative. While they contain large amounts of protein and starchy materials, they are very poor in the positive mineral salts, and what little they possess of these important elements is stored in the germ, pericarp and in the dark outer layers. In order to comply with the popular demand for white flour and white rice, these outer layers are removed in the milling processes, and thus grains and rice are robbed of their most valuable blood and bone making elements, as well as of the vitamins. Bran and rice polishings are, therefore, exceedingly rich in mineral salts and are very valuable foods for our domestic animals. The latter wax strong and fat on the "refuse" of the mills — rich in organic salts — while the farmer grows thin and dyspeptic on his fine white flour. As long as oriental nations used unpolished rice, which is richer in flavour as well as better fitted to sustain life than is our refined but impoverished mill product, they remained immune to beriberi and similar diseases. We have already explained how the refining and polishing robs the grains and rice of their mineral elements and vitamins.

Conclusions

Let us see whether, after this brief survey of our food tables, we can explain some of the mysteries and perplexities of dietetics. We can understand now why our American vegetarians, living largely on devitalized leguminous and grain products, with a liberal allowance of nuts, peanuts and olive oil, often fare worse than people living on a mixed diet, and become "warning examples" to meat eaters. A look at the mineral constituents of grain and rice answers most effectively the common argument of the anti-vegetarian: "Look at your vegetarian nations in the orient, the Hindus and Chinese. Would you lower us to their physical and mental level by the adoption of a vegetarian diet?" Grains and rice rank lowest in the scale of negative foods, and it is therefore no wonder that people living almost exclusively on these staples should be subnormal, physically and mentally. Also highly dangerous to those who are already negative and sensitive is a straight raw food, or fruit and nut diet. It is only a naturally very positive "animal" constitution that can afford to live on such a negative and highly refining diet. Many fruit-and-nut enthusiasts expressly exclude from their dietary all things growing in and under the ground, as well as the dairy products, "because they are coarsening and tend to develop the animal nature." In their endeavour to make short cuts to masterhood and godhood, by the diet route, they forget that in these strenuous, physical-material surroundings we need a considerable amount of the positive animal magnetic qualities in our daily business. In fact, negative food combinations and excessive fasting can lead misguided idealists and enthusiasts into physical and mental breakdown and into abnormal psychism, obsession and insanity. This is especially so when they fall under the influence of fake occultists or spiritual advisers who encourage them in undesirable forms of meditation, and subjective psychism.

A rational vegetarian diet properly combined, consisting of dairy products, the positive vegetables and medium positive fruits, with just enough starchy and protein foods to supply the needs of the body for tissue building and fuel materials, will be found to be an ideal diet, fully sufficient to sustain health and strength in the most trying circumstances.

We admit that there are cases of physical and nervous breakdown in which magnetic conditions have become so negative that a meat diet is, temporarily, of great advantage to supply the lack of animal magnetism. The animal magnetism derived from flesh foods is, however, only borrowed, and is contaminated by the poisonous waste matter of the dead animal carcas. Therefore we have seen people cured of negative mental conditions by the Salisbury raw meat diet, only to develop rheumatism, heart disease, calculi in kidneys and bladder, and other uric acid diseases. Natural Therapeutics follows a wiser plan. By its stimulating methods of natural treatment and eliminating, yet positive, vegetarian diet, it puts the organism of the patient in such a condition that it can generate its own positive magnetic energies([1]).

([1])
The Analytical Food Table in this chapter deals only with the thirteen most important elements found in the human body. However, research has led to the discovery of seventeen or more elements in the body though some of these exist only in very small amounts. It is certain that all or most of them are useful or essential for the life or health of the body, and in the case of some of them, such as copper, iodine and zinc, at least something is known of the functions which they perform. Since all these elements should be furnished by food the question of their supply is linked with the condition of the soil and the presence in it of everything which is required to support plant and animal life. This is a vindication of the emphasis which Lindlahr lays on the importance of maintaining the proper mineralization of the soil. Some modern research has established that the presence or absence in the soil of minute quantities of some trace element, such as boron, may make the difference between a useful fertility and a useless barrenness.

CHAPTER XIX

MISCELLANEOUS

The Psychology of Digestion

All we can do is to give the general outlines of food selection; the details and individual application must be worked out personally. No two organisms are just alike, and their requirements of food and drink differ in quantity and quality from day to day, especially in times of healing crises, under natural treatment. As the system changes, as the morbid materials are eliminated and new and normal tissues are elaborated, the demands of the organism for certain food elements constantly change. Always, however, they keep within the well defined limits of natural food selection. For weeks a patient may live almost entirely on celery and cabbage slaws, then he may develop a craving for tomatoes or carrots; again he may exhibit a strong desire for certain fruits or nuts. We always advise our patients to satisfy these cravings, which are especially peculiar to pregnancy and to periods of healing crises. They usually indicate a special need of the system for certain elements contained in these foods.

Caprice and false appetite, however, must not be mistaken for natural craving, and even the latter should not be encouraged nor satisfied continually unless it falls within the limits of natural food selection. Frequently, when we outline our system of dietetics to a new patient he exclaims in horror: "Why, I cannot possibly eat this or that; it would kill me", or the complaint is: "I like those vegetables, but they do not like me; they cause great distress. Must I eat them in spite of this?" "No", we answer, "if such is the case, do not use them for the present; you probably will use them after a while. Select at first within the right limits, those fruits and vegetables which agree with you. As your digestive organs become more normal you will add to your dietary, one after another, the luscious fruits and vegetables which now invariably cause pain, noxious gases and other symptoms of fermentation and indigestion".

Present disease conditions were caused by a lack of these foods and the organic salts which they contain. A permanent cure can be produced only by the gradual adoption of the acid solving and acid binding foods, even if, temporarily, they create a commotion in the heavily encumbered organs and tissues. A thorough house cleaning makes the dirt fly, stirs the poisons from their hiding places, throws them into circulation and brings them in contact with the living tissues, thus producing the acute aggravations of healing crises. But as we cannot have a clean house to live in without an occasional scouring so we cannot have a clean body without an occasional healing crisis. When you begin to live on a natural diet, never mind the unpleasant disturbances, the capricious and alternating diarrhoeas and constipations; they all belong to the game of house cleaning and renovating.

These changes and crises in the physical body are usually accompanied by more or less mental depression, irritability and melancholia. The old things are passing away and the new are coming in. It is the vastation of the old and the generation of the new man. Hence the queer feeling of "goneness", of "being lost" and "homesickness" so often described by our patients in times of healing crises.

Idiosyncrasies

Idiosyncrasies are habits of body and mind peculiar to an individual. Most individuals exhibit some idiosyncracy in connection with food. They cannot eat certain wholesome foods; one cannot eat an apple, another has an abhorrence for bread, still another becomes nauseated when eating sweets. Some of these peculiar traits are congenital and due to prenatal influences; others are caused by eating too much or too often of a certain kind of food. Sometimes they are due to mental or psychic neuroses; in other instances disease conditions in the body revolt against a certain food and create an idiosyncrasy. Whatever the cause of these annoying dislikes and antipathies they can be overcome by improving the general condition of the organism, particularly the digestive organs, and by autosuggestion.[1] Every evening before falling asleep, dwell upon the thought that the particular food which in the

[1]
    It is a remarkable thing that the word "allergy" does not appear in any of Lindlahr's writings. In these days, however, allergies have assumed a great importance and have become a great preoccupation of many physicians. Many patients are tested for allergies or are believed to have them and some such patients are reduced to a condition in which it becomes extremely difficult to know what is left for them to eat. In Lindlahr's view when a patient appears to react unfavourably to foods which are natural and healthy and which are good from a dietetic point of view, it means that the trouble is in the patient and not in the food. Sometimes such reactions and antipathies are due to mental or psychological causes and can be got rid of by autosuggestion, but in any case the problem is not to be solved by taking the patient off good foods to which he reacts unfavourably, except possibly for a short time, but by improving his digestion and re-educating his tastes so that he tolerates them and derives pleasure and benefit from them. Indeed it must be remembered that in some cases when a food produces reactions such as diarrhoea or skin eruptions it means that it is bringing about a very useful elimination and is in fact needed by the body. There are, however, some idiosyncrasies or allergies which would appear to be so built into the constitutions of certain people that they cannot tolerate certain foods and will become seriously ill if they do not abstain from them, and in the case of children, will not develop normally if they are given them. The most outstanding example of this is so-called "coeliac disease" which is an intolerance to all foods containing gluten derived from cereals such as wheat, rye and oats and for which the only remedy would appear to be to put the patient onto a gluten-free diet which, it is now thought, may have to be continued throughout life. Information about gluten-free diets is readily available.

past has annoyed or distressed you, henceforth will perfectly agree with you. Say to yourself: "It is a good wholesome food; it contains valuable elements of nutrition which I need in the economy of my body. There is no reason why I should not eat it. I will not allow my subconsious mind to tyrannize over my waking consciousness. I am master of my feelings and my actions and not the plaything of prenatal influence, foolish fear or morbid suggestion. I am master of my body, mind and soul."

Mental Dyspepsia

Many people spoil the beneficial effects of the natural food regimen by excessive anxiety. No matter how good the advice and how carefully they follow it, they are always in fear of making mistakes about this food or that, of eating too much or eating too little; they ponder every morsel and worry over it; then for a day or two they analyze their symptoms and try to determine how this dish of gruel or that bit of cheese affected them. Such a mental attitude is weakening and destructive; it will poison the most wholesome food and drink. Mental dyspepsia will inevitably express itself in physical indigestion and malnutrition. To the best of your ability, make your food selection: so much of the organic salt group, so much of protein and so much of carbohydrates. When an understanding of the rudiments of food chemistry has been acquired, the right selections are made without trouble and almost intuitively. When the food is on the table, forget the problems of dietetics, put all thought of business, work and study far from you and centre your attention on pleasant things, and the joy of eating. With every morsel duly masticated, swallow a happy thought or a pleasant emotion. Build castles in the air, be merry, have a friendly word and a happy smile for wife and child or for your chance acquaintance at the table d'hote.

The medieval court jester, whose office it was to amuse the guests at a feast or banquet, was a sensible and useful institution, much more worthy of patronage than poisonous pills and tonics. Worry, anxiety, anger, hatred and peevishness contract the blood vessels, inhibit the flow of digestive fluids as well as the mental disposition. On the other hand, nothing stimulates the circulation and the flow of gastric juices, or sweetens the secretions, like cheerfulness, happiness and absolute confidence in the healing power within. If by chance you have made a mistake or committed an indiscretion in eating, do not make it worse by worrying over it. Take a good big dose of mental-magic tonic, one hundred grains of courage well shaken in a few ounces of cheerfulness,

96

thereby increasing the flow of gastric secretions and say to yourself: "Since I have eaten the forbidden fruit, I will not worry over it; my innate powers of body, mind and soul will neutralize the bad effects. I will appropriate the good there is in it and eliminate the evil". Use forethought and self control to avoid mistakes, but when you have made one do not make matters worse by fearthought.

Over-Eating

The most wholesome food becomes injurious when taken in excessive quantities. Whatever we cannot properly digest and assimilate ferments and decays filling the system with waste matter and poison. Many persons squander their vitality in eliminating noxious food ballast, and wonder why they are so weak in spite of good appetite and rich foods. When the organs of digestion are continually overworked they weaken and become unable to convert the oversupply of food into the proper constituents for healthy blood and lymph; waste matter accumulates, creating noxious gases and systemic poisons. Poisonous miasms thus contaminate the vital fluids, causing corruption and obstruction in organs and tissues, and furnishing a luxurious soil for the growth of all kinds of parasites, germs and bacteria.

In chapters III and IV it was shown that one cannot eat and drink vital force since it is independent of food, drink, medicine and tonics. It is hard to comprehend why so many physicians persist in stuffing the weak bodies of consumptives and other invalids with enormous quantities of food, under the mistaken impression that the patients can thus be strengthened and improved in health. Is it not self-evident that the stomachs of these poor sufferers are as feeble and incapable of exertion as their arms and legs? If they were able properly to digest and assimilate even a few eggs a day they would not be so weak and emaciated, but in spite of their weakened condition they are "stuffed" with as many eggs as they can possibly force down their throats. The result is that the entire mass decays and ferments, spoiling that which was necessary together with the superfluous, thus doing more harm than good to the body. Is it not more sensible to give no more than the digestive organs can take care of, and gradually to increase the amount of food as stomach and intestines become more active and alive under natural methods of treatment?

Fasting Imperative in Acute Diseases

In serious diseases, and in states of nervous and physical prostration, the expenditure of vital force is at a minimum, as is apparent from the extreme weakness and helplessness of the patient; therefore, much less food is required than in times of healthful activity. Does not nature herself protest against eating by loss of appetite, nausea and vomiting? Nevertheless, though the patient himself objects to the enforced feeding, and his whole organism revolts against it, doctor and friends insist that he "must eat to keep up strength". "Sedatives" are given to paralyse the stomach into submission and down go chicken soup, eggs, beef tea and other tempting morsels.

In acute febrile diseases, feeding is not only useless but actually harmful, because in such conditions the normal activities of the organism, including the processes of digestion and assimilation, are at a standstill. All efforts are concentrated on elimination, the stomach and bowels being called upon to assist in the general house cleaning. Instead of assimilating, they, too, are eliminating noxious poisons which produce nausea, vomiting, diarrhoea and catarrhal excretions. The digestive organs normally act like a sponge — they absorb the food elements from the digestive tract and transmit them into the blood stream. In febrile diseases the process is reversed — the sponge is being squeezed. It is throwing off morbid excretions, thus aiding the cleansing crisis. As soon as food is given, this beneficial elimination through stomach and bowels is hindered and interrupted; as a consequence, the temperature rises and aggravation of all symptoms follows. The danger lies not so much in under-feeding as in over-feeding. To one who dies from lack of food, thousands die from over-eating. If the truth were known we should be surprised at the small amount of food required to keep the body in perfect condition.

Cornaro, an Italian nobleman, when forty years of age, was declared by his doctors to be dying from the effects of dissipation. Instead of resigning himself to his fate, he determined to enter upon an experiment of his own. He cut his food supply down to twelve ounces a day, and, before long, regained health and strength. At a hundred years of age he wrote a book in which he describes his experiences and the wonderful effects of temperate living. When about eighty years of age, Cornaro felt for a while somewhat indisposed. His relatives and friends at once overwhelmed him with reproaches, saying that he was weakening and killing himself by slow starvation. In compliance with their entreaties, he increased his food allowance by a few ounces a day, but this affected him so badly that he was forced to return to his customary allowance.

The only safe guide in eating is hunger, not appetite. True hunger is nature's sign that more food is needed, and that the organism is in a condition to take care of it. If these simple truths were more widely understood and patients in acute disease were fasted instead of stuffed the death rate would decrease to an astonishing degree.

To Salt or Not to Salt?

Like Banquo's ghost this question will not lie down. Pro or con it has been discussed by every diet specialist and food reformer. Vegetarians say: "Don't", meat eaters say: "Do". Both may be right, but how can that be? Common inorganic table salt is chemically composed of sodium and chlorine. We call sodium and all other minerals organic when they have entered into chemical combinations with carbon or protein compounds in the living cells of plants and animals. We have learned in other chapters of this volume that potatoes, fats and sugars in the process of digestion form large amounts of poisonous acids, alkaloids and ptomaines, which become a most fruitful source of disease when not rapidly and thoroughly eliminated. The neutralization and elimination of these food poisons depend largely upon sodium. The ordinary American diet, consisting of meats, peas, beans, potatoes, white bread, pastry, coffee and sugar, contains an excessive amount of the acid producing food elements, and only very small amounts of the eliminating sodium. Fruits and vegetables, however, are very rich in organic sodium as well as all other positive alkaline mineral elements. Keeping in mind these premises, we see how both vegetarian and meat eater may be right in their stands on the salt question. The vegetarian, whose daily dietary contains a liberal amount of uncooked fruits and vegetables and only moderate amounts of proteins and starches, has no need and no desire for inorganic table salt. His demands for sodium are fully satisfied in a natural way by the organic sodium contained in the raw foods. On the other hand, people whose dietary consists largely of meats, potatoes, peas, beans, cereal foods, white flour bread and pastry, coffee, tea and refined sugar, all of which are lacking in the acid binding sodium, must have salt in order to make up the deficiency of this element in their food — therefore, they have a strong craving for the inorganic table salt.

The foods above mentioned, as we have learned, produce large amounts of poisonous acids and alkaloids, and unless these are promptly neutralized and eliminated by sodium, disease and death would be the inevitable results. Since the above described American dietary is deficient in the organic salts of fruits and vegetables, inorganic table salt (sodium chloride) must serve as a poor substitute, but it is far better for the system to have the inorganic substitute than no sodium at all. The fact that many people have lived almost entirely on meats or cereal foods with table salt as seasoning, and have reached a ripe old age, indicates that the organism can use the inorganic salt as a substitute for the organic.

We have learned that many elements, though congenial to the body, when taken in inorganic form show in the iris, but table salt, even when habitually taken in large quantities, does not show, indicating that we cannot class it among the poison foods. It is congenial to the system, being naturally present in the blood in organic combinations, in considerable quantities. Like uric acid, caffeine, theine, alcohol and nicotine, which also do not show in the iris by distinct signs, it becomes injurious to the system only when taken habitually in large quantities. Possibly table salt stands in closer relationship to the vito-chemical life element than the mineral substances which show in the iris. Table salt, however, should be used very moderately, even by meat eaters. Its excessive use easily becomes a habit. Its elimination greatly irritates the kidneys and withdraws from the blood large quantities of serum. This creates thirst, which necessitates the drinking of much water. This in turn dilutes the blood and other secretions of the organism, causing a watery dysaemia of all the vital fluids.

Our flushing faddists seem to regard an excess of water in blood and tissues as a desirable condition — our farmers know how to turn this into money. Salt, given to cattle and hogs, creates abnormal thirst. This causes excessive water drinking and watery dysaemia (anaemia); watery blood makes fat. Thus salt is turned into fat and fat into money. Inorganic salt, when absorbed in large quantities, pickles the tissues. It destroys albuminous compounds and causes their excessive secretion in the urine (albuminuria). Therefore, it leeches the protoplasm of the cells, weakening their resistance and breaking down their normal structures. This is shown clearly in scurvy, which is caused by the excessive use of salt meats and the lack of fresh vegetables with their organic salts and vitamins. This disease, which is characterised by decay and bleeding of the gums, proves that nature limits the substitution of inorganic salt for the organic, and it strongly indicates that the organic is the most desirable form. As soon as scurvy patients are put on a fruit and vegetable diet, the destruction of tissues, the bleeding resulting from it and other symptoms promptly abate.

Another indication that inorganic sodium chloride is not congenial to the system is indicated by the fact that considerable amounts of the organic salt contained in fruits and vegetables or in their extracts do not create thirst, while comparatively small amounts of the inorganic table salts cause irritation and over work of the kidneys, great thirst, albuminuria, and weakening of the cell structure. These influences undoubtedly favour the development of kidney diseases.

Now that we have considered the evidence for and against the use of salt, we shall endeavour to answer the question. Is it advisable for vegetarians to use salt? When the dietary contains liberal amounts of uncooked fruits and vegetables, very little or no salt will be needed. The addition of salt is permissible to vegetarian foods which contain large amounts of proteins, fats and starches, such as eggs, butter, peas, beans, lentils, potatoes, cereals and rice. Vegetables of the fifth group when properly steamed in their own juices so that none of their mineral constituents are wasted, do not need additional condiments; their own salts are the best flavouring.[2]

In conclusion we must remember that fruits and vegetables often do not contain the normal amounts of organic salts, because for ages the soil on which they have grown has been robbed of its mineral constituents. It is this deficiency in mineral elements which lowers the resistance of vegetables, grains and fruits, impairs their development, causes decay and facilitates the work of destructive worms, insects and germs, just as lowered resistance and lack of vitamins favours the development of germs and bacteria in human bodies. Nitrogenous fertilizers have been provided plentifully, but the necessity of positive mineral fertilizers was never thought of until Julius Hensel, the Nature Cure

[2]
Sodium does undoubtedly play a very important part in the economy of the body. However, it is not present in sufficient quantities in some soils and consequently may be lacking in the food grown in such soils. According to Lindlahr this deficiency can be made up to some extent by the use of inorganic table salt, but to use much of it is harmful, and the proper way to provide sodium is to apply small quantities of rock salt to the land. Of recent years there have been many who maintain that, in so far as salt is used it should not be the pure sodium chloride which is generally sold commercially, but should be sea salt or specially prepared biochemic salt which contains other minerals as well and can be regarded as being more natural and better balanced. This is a view which would seem to have a sound basis as there is evidence that there is danger in the chemical balance of the body being upset, in particular the sodium-potassium balance.

Lindlahr, in common with others who think along homoeopathic lines, is undoubtedly right in pointing out the danger to health in the very lavish and immoderate use of salt which is common in many homes and restaurants, both in the kitchens and at table. Salt has a hardening effect on the arteries by reducing their elasticity and so causing high blood pressure. It is probably conducive to the formation of cataract. It holds fluid in the tissues and so can contribute to weight increase which in turn can put a strain on the heart. Also it irritates the kidneys and appears to inhibit their proper functioning, especially as heavy salt users have an abnormal thirst and take in large quantities of fluid. Excessive sodium tends to be excreted through the skin and the sinuses and therefore salt should be avoided by people suffering from skin and sinus troubles.

The fact that salt is much excreted through the skin led, during the last war, to the idea that the troops serving in the tropics were in danger of suffering from sodium deficiency and they were heavily dosed with salt to counteract the loss of sodium. Except in some very exceptional circumstances the giving of a lot of extra salt in this way is harmful rather than beneficial because people in the tropics and elswhere do not require extra salt if they have a good diet with plenty of fruit and vetetables, and when they have eliminated excess salt they cease to excrete it through the skin. The idea that giving salt is a good treatment for cramp would also seem to be erroneous. Muscle cramps are usually a sign that the muscles in question are in a hard contracted condition which causes them to go into a painful spasm and not to relax normally when they should. This condition can be changed by deep massage of the muscles.

food chemist, called attention to the fact. The soil and its products, therefore, as well as human beings, suffer from mineral starvation and deficiency of vitamins. African explorers state that in certain parts of Africa the soil and its products are lacking in sodium chloride, and that in these sections animals and human beings suffer from salt starvation, which expresses itself in many ways.

The addition of small quantities of table salt to a vegetarian diet is, therefore, not to be condemned, but its use should generally be confined to butter, eggs and such cooked foods as we have mentioned. Do not use it at the table, except on eggs. It is barbaric to kill with salt and pepper the delicate flavours of fruits and vegetables. "But", says our friend, the meat eater, "I have to add condiments and spice, or I cannot taste anything". To this we answer: "No wonder, when the taste buds in your tongue are paralyzed by salt, pepper, mustard, strong condiments, nicotine and alcohol. Return to a natural diet and your nerves of taste will soon regain their natural sensitiveness. Then you will enjoy the delicious flavours of fruits and vegetables, and things will taste as good as 'when mother made them' ".

Fermented Bread

It has been the habit of vegetarians to condemn the use of fermented bread. They have usually given as the reasons for this the following arguments:
(1) That fermented bread contains yeast germs, which cause injurious fermentation in the digestive tract; (2) that fermented bread contains alcohol, which is injurious to health and life; (3) that the "raising" of the dough is due to gases arising from the decaying bodies of dead yeast germs; (4) that the transformation of the sugar in the fermenting dough entails a considerable loss of elements of nutrition. None of these objections seems in fact to have any real validity. As regards (1) it is well established that yeast germs die at a temperature of about 150 degrees Fahrenheit. It is therefore most unlikely that any of them would survive the heat of a bake oven. If any of them should do so it would not be a matter of great moment. Physiology teaches us that the various processes of digestion are completed in the intestinal tract by germ fermentation. That is to say that while digestion is initiated by the enzymes such as ptyalin, pepsin and the pancreatic ferments, it is carried on and completed by fungi and bacteria of many kinds in the intestinal tract. Many of these organisms are of the yeast type and the addition of a few yeast germs can do no harm and may even do good seeing that all the processes of digestion are, in a way, processes of

fermentation. As regards (2) it may be true that very small quantities of alcohol may be formed in fermented bread as is revealed by chemical tests, but there is not enough of it left in the bread to do harm of any kind. Indeed alcohol is naturally produced in the healthy human body to a certain extent by the oxidation of food materials and waste matter. It is, therefore, in small quantities, congenial to the system and plays a useful part in the vital activities and it does not become dangerous to health and life unless present in excessive quantities. Alcohol is easily combustible and acts as fuel material to the system. When present in large quantities, however, it paralyses the inhibitory nervous apparatus and burns up nerve fats too rapidly, thereby causing temporary over-stimulation and resultant weakness and exhaustion. As regards (3) it may be said that dead yeast germs have never been known to create carbonic acid gas in considerable quantities. They have to be alive in order to do so. Yeast fungi, while living on sugar, digest or split up the sugar into alcohol and carbonic acid gas. This gas, while escaping, per-meates the dough with air passages and bubbles and in that way raises and lightens it. This loosening of the dough into a sponge-like mass favours the escape of moisture and the penetration of heat. The result-ing bread is therefore baked more thoroughly and keeps much better, does not sour so quickly, and is more easily digested than much of the soggy, lumpy, "unfermented health bread". This carbonic acid gas which lightens the bread cannot be very injurious. When taken as a free gas into the stomach in food or drink, it rapidly evaporates, and while escaping creates that cooling, prickling and refreshing sensation peculiar to carbonated beverages. As regards (4) it may be said that the loss of sugar incidental to bread fermentation is so small that it hardly merits consideration. This small loss is more than balanced by increased digestibility and palatableness and by better keeping qual-ities

What has been said will make it apparent that the fermentation of the bread is, in a way, a process of predigestion. In fact, all so called predigested health foods have been subjected to some process of fer-mentation, for in this way only is it possible to "predigest" food materials. This, however, is not altogether an advantage. Predigestion dissipates, outside of the body, food energy which should be liberated and utilized inside the body.

Mono-Diet

One of the latest developments in dietetic treatment is the mono-diet. Strictly speaking, this regimen consists in taking but one article of food at a meal, a succession of meals, or continuously for a considerable period of time. The mono-diet, like the grape cure, milk cure, raw food diet, Salisbury raw meat diet, fasting, Fletcherizing, and other forms of radical and one-sided dietetic treatment, when applied temporarily, may have very beneficial effects on certain diseased conditions, and for the attainment of special results. But it is not advisable to prescribe or to follow an extreme regimen indiscriminately, in all kinds of cases, or for indefinite periods of time. The trouble is that enthusiasts look upon such methods as cure-alls, apply them to all kinds of cases and conditions, and thereby often inflict lasting injuries upon those who entrust themselves to their care. Because these extreme practices are beneficial in some cases, their advocates jump to the conclusion that they will prove efficacious in all circumstances. One of the principal objections to the mono-diet is that not one article of food, with the exception of milk and red blood, contains, in right proportions, all the elements required by the body. All the foods of the first four groups as shown in our tables of food analysis (pages 84 and 85) contain too much of the negative acid-forming elements and not enough of the positive mineral salts and vitamins, while the foods of the fifth group contain enough of the positive mineral elements, but not enough of the heating and building materials. Any extreme, one-sided diet, therefore, must in the long run necessarily lead to unbalanced and abnormal conditions in the system. Furthermore, mono-diet means monotony, and monotony in eating, as in many other things, is not conducive to health, happiness and longevity. We naturally crave variety in our foods as well as in our surroundings and occupations. Mono-tony — sameness of tone — is not harmony; therefore not pleasing; and if long continued, becomes annoying and destructive. Desire for food and the keen enjoyment of it depend upon a moderate variety at least. Keen appetite and hunger ensure copious secretion of the digestive juices and ferments. One often hears people say that they cannot eat a certain food because at one time they "ate too much of it". Frequently we are told by patients of a revulsion to a particular perfectly wholesome and inviting food which has been acquired in this way and this confirms us in our opinion that a mono-diet is not natural.([3]).

However, in many cases where we have had to counteract a certain form of systemic poisoning, we have found the mono-diet very benefi-

---

([3]) Experiments on animals have confirmed that the digestive juices of dogs flow more freely when they are confronted with food which they like than when they are shown food to which they are indifferent or which they do not like. Also the secretions of animals excited to fear or anger are greatly diminished.

cial, as, for instance, the grape cure or the milk cure in uric acid diseases. In such cases the mono-diet constitutes a mild form of protein starvation, which is desirable for a time in the circumstances. On the other hand, when patients are already physically and mentally weak and inactive, have lost ambition and energy together with appetite, all such extremes as fasting, raw food diet and mono-diet may become positively harmful and lead to nervous prostration, abnormal psychism and insanity. No radical or extreme form of diet or other method of treatment should ever be undertaken except under the advice and guidance of a competent physician, who is capable of taking into consideration the various aspects and requirements of the case.(⁴)

Mastication

Thorough mastication of food is an absolute necessity to insure good digestion, but, like every other good thing, can be overdone. Horace Fletcher, in his *A-B-C of Nutrition*, advocates mastication of food until it is reduced to a fluid condition. While I believe that Fletcherizing has benefited many people suffering from overeating and consequent food poisoning, I know also that in many instances it has been positively harmful. Food in a liquid state does not offer enough resistance to the muscles of the intestinal tract. Stomach and intestines need some bulky, solid food as a stimulus to peristalsis, the propelling movement peculiar to the digestive organs. If all food be converted into a liquid before it enters the stomach, the peristaltic movements of the digestive tract will become ineffective through disuse and the bowels will become lazy and inactive as they do under a milk diet. Furthermore, most people simply cannot afford the time to Fletcherize. To do this would require an hour or more each meal. Instead of spending this time at the table trying to reduce the cellulose and woody fibre of fruits and vegetables to a liquid, thereby destroying their stimulating effect upon the stomach and intestines, it would be much more beneficial to take fifteen to thirty minutes after each meal for relaxation, rest and

(⁴) While Lindlahr's criticism of mono-diets in general is no doubt sound, it would appear that the grape cure has someting very special to offer, and can be used successfully in very grave conditions, including malignancy, when all other measures have failed. This would seem to be because grape juice is a wonderful purifier and is also so easy to assimilate that it puts no tax on the digestion and does not interfere with elimination. In fact, it provides an exception to the general rule that the body cannot readily assimilate and eliminate, build up and break down at the same time. This makes the grape cure an alternative to starvation in cases where the body is too weak to sustain a long fast or to benefit by it. The uses and possibilities of the grape cure are discussed in books by Johanna Brandt and Basil Shackleton (Thorson's).

It also appears that some patients with digestive troubles get on better if they are given one kind of food only at one meal.

vital regeneration. This is specially to be recommended to people with very weak digestions. When they are thoroughly relaxed and at rest they should, by an effort of will, concentrate the blood and nerve currents on the work of the digestive organs.

Frequency of Meals

The frequency of meals cannot be determined by hard and fast rules. Different factors must be taken into account — occupation, physical condition, the circumstances in the home, and so forth. As a rule the two-meal plan is the best. The ideal way is to have breakfast between nine and ten o'clock in the morning and dinner between five and six in the afternoon. This allows sufficient time for thorough digestion and assimilation. In our experience, the no-breakfast plan does not agree with most people. Putting off the first meal until noon is likely to create excessive hunger and a tendency to overeat. If circumstances are such that breakfast has to be taken early in the day and dinner late in the evening, it may be found advisable to eat a light lunch at noon, consisting of fruit and a few nuts; or a vegetable salad; or some whole grain bread and a glass of milk. Some of our friends and patients get along best on one meal a day. This is especially advisable where there is a tendency to over-eating and to excessive fat and flesh formation. In certain cases of an exceptionally weak and negative condition we have found it expedient to give small quantities of food three or four times a day.

Drinking

We are not in favour of excessive drinking. The "flushing of the system" fad is a mistake. The purification of the body is not a mechanical process like the flushing of a sewer with water. It is a chemical process which depends upon the normal composition and concentration of the different secretions in the system. These secretions, the most important one of which is the blood, cannot be made more effective by diluting them with large amounts of water. Most of the people suffering from stubborn chronic constipation who come to us for treatment have been "flushing" for years, through mouth and rectum, with the result that they were getting more constipated all the time. On our comparatively dry food diet the bowels, in most cases, begin to act normally within a short time. Dry food stimulates the secretions of the intestines. Constant flushing makes them more lazy and inactive. Furthermore, much of the water saturated with poisonous accumulations in the rectum and colon is reabsorbed into the system.

It is the customary highly spiced meat and egg diet which creates excessive and abnormal thirst. A rational non-irritating and non-stimulating vegetarian diet furnishes the organism with fluids of the best possible kind in the form of fruit and vegetable juices, prepared in nature's own laboratory, rich in medicinal qualities and free from all objectionable constituents. Under ordinary conditions, drink from four to eight glasses of pure water of ordinary temperature in the course of the day, according to your own individual inclination; in the morning before breakfast, at night before going to bed, and at intervals during the day. (⁵)

Distilled Water

Another popular fallacy is the idea that on account of its absolute purity distilled water is wholesome. As a matter of fact, its very purity makes it injurious to the system. All water has a natural tendency to saturate itself, up to a certain point, with mineral matter. Good drinking water always contains a certain amount of mineral matter. When this is removed through distillation, the water will leech from the system the organic mineral salts which play such an important part in the vital processes of our bodies, and which we find it is so difficult to supply in sufficient amounts. Good drinking water is agreeable to the taste, whereas the absence of mineral salts accounts for the flat taste of distilled water.

On the other hand, very large quantities of lime, iron, sulphur, or other inorganic minerals in water that is used constantly for drinking or bathing, are injurious to the system If such minerals are present in excess, the water should be boiled and allowed to settle before it is used. It may be oxygenated and revitalized by passing through it a mild current of electricity. If the water contains vegetable or animal organic matter it should be filtered.

Drinking at Meals

The less you drink with your meals the better. The dryness of the

---

(⁵) Lindlahr definitely ranges himself on the side of those who do not believe in too much drinking, and no doubt he is right in condemning the radical "flushing" treatment which has sometimes been favoured by some practitioners of the Nature Cure school. On the other hand, it would appear that there are now many who go to the other extreme and who discourage their patients from drinking enough or even at all. While it is true that people well established on a strict vegetarian diet can get along well drinking very little indeed, it would seem that in a general way people drink too little rather than too much, especially if they are not strict vegetarians on a good vegetarian diet. Lindlahr's actual prescription of from four to eight glasses of water or dilute fruit juice per day is not ungenerous as this represents two to four pints. It appears that sometimes at the start of treatment good results are obtained by giving more than this for a short time to reduce a condition of marked toxicity. All would appear to be agreed that there should be little or no drinking at meals.

food furnishes the necessary stimulus to the secretion of saliva and gastric and intestinal juices. An abundance of liquid in the digestive tract interferes with the action of the secreting glands. Moreover, it dilutes the secretions and thereby weakens their digestive qualities. The juices of the stomach and the intestines cannot be made more effective by adding to them large quantities of water at meal times. Coffee and tea or alcoholic drinks should especially be avoided at meals. The former retard digestion; the latter overstimulate temporarily the secretion of gastric and intestinal juices, and this unnatural stimulation is followed by corresponding weakness and inactivity of the secreting glands in the digestive tract. Liquor taken before and during meals, therefore, encourages over-eating, and when the reaction sets in, the secretions as well as the vitality are lacking in strength to digest properly the excess of food taken under the influence of unnatural stimulation. A glass of water taken from thirty to sixty minutes before meals will, in most cases, do away with the desire to drink at meal times. However, if there is actual thirst, it must be satisfied, especially when the digestive juices of the stomach are over-charged with acids. In that case a glass of cool water will reduce hyperacidity. Never use iced water. If you prefer a warm drink you may take cereal coffee, or warm milk, or (sparingly) cocoa. Skimmed milk, buttermilk and fruit juices diluted with water are good cold drinks.

Mixing Starches with Acid Fruits and Vegetables

Many dietists lay great stress on the idea that acid fruit juices retard or prevent the digestion of starchy foods in the stomach. Therefore, they advise that these foods should never be taken at the same meal. We find that this rule does not hold good in all cases. It is true that some people cannot eat starchy foods and acids at the same meal, without experiencing serious digestive disturbances and aggravation of chronic symptoms. This is especially true of those who suffer with hyperacidity of the stomach and catarrhal ailments. The latter are frequently caused by starch poisoning, due to putrefying starchy materials in the digestive tract. On the other hand, most of our patients do not experience any bad effects from the mixing of starches with fruit and vegetable acids. This is especially true of those who incline to hyperacidity, and who take good care thoroughly to masticate and insalivate the starchy foods before they swallow them. Thus it is that while with some people fruit and vegetable acids seem to increase the acidity of the stomach, with a great many others they antidote acidity. To those who belong to this class, acid fruit is the best cure. We know of such people suffering from acidity of the stomach in the middle of the night, arising to eat a few oranges. Relief and sleep soon follow. The alkaline elements of juicy fruits neutralize the hyperacidity of the stomach and the blood. However, in all cases where the mixing of these foods causes the least trouble, it certainly should be avoided. Such people should take with their cereals, sweet alkaline fruits only, such as dates, figs, raisins, stewed prunes, sweet grapes and melons in season. They should take the acid fruits by themselves, for the noonday lunch, or if they have the heavy meal of the day at noon, they should have nothing but acid fruits or vegetables for breakfast, or between breakfast and dinner at noon.[6]

The acid fruits and vegetables may be taken together with dairy products, fats or protein foods, such as milk, buttermilk, cream, cheese, honey, eggs, meat and nuts. The acid foods should be avoided at the heavy meal consisting of starches, fats, proteins and alkaline vegetables.

[6] Lindlahr attributes the origin of the idea that starches should not be mixed with acid fruits and vegetables to a certain Dr. I. H. Tilden who was a well-known writer on Natural Dietetics at that time. He also attributes to Tilden the origin of the theory that copious water drinking is a good cure for constipation. In both cases, however, Tilden appears to have changed his mind and to have recanted these opinions in his later writings. Some modern writers on dietetics, however, still lay very great stress on the dangers of mixing foods regarded as incompatible in the digestive tract. This idea is developed very forcibly and in great detail by the French naturopath, Robert Masson, in his works "Soignex-vous par la Nature" and "Folie et Sagesse des Médicines Naturelles". These books are interesting and impressive and are worthy of careful study. In some respects his views and methods are in accord with those of Lindlahr but there are a number of points of disagreement and differences of emphasis. It is difficult not to feel that some of his ideas and assertions, if not actually erroneous, are exaggerated or of limited applicability, though he supports them with many interesting case reports from his own experience. Certain foods or mixtures of foods are condemned altogether or deprecated as being difficult to digest. In particular, he lays great emphasis on the undesirability of mixing starches and fruits (especially acid fruits) because the digestion of the former can be inhibited in the mouth and stomach and, as a result, the digestive tract can become filled with undigested material which ferments, causing gas formation, malassimilation and catarrhal conditions, notably of the respiratory tract. He is also critical of the numerous rigid systems of diet which have been or are being followed by many diet reformers. He discusses some of these systems and points out the possible dangers and weaknesses of each. Altogether he is opposed to too much rigidity and dogmatism in matters of diet. To him, it would seem, the things of real importance are that the foods eaten should not be denatured or added to in processing, especially by the use of chemicals or preservatives, that alcohol, tea, coffee, tobacco and other toxins should be avoided and that overeating, especially of starches and fats, so very prevalent now in western countries, should be discouraged. The actual dietary regimen prescribed in a particular case should be very much individualised to the patient's requirements and should be influenced and determined by such things as age, climate and way of life. It is interesting to note that many of the prescriptions which are given for the treatment of particular diseases or conditions make use of traditional French tisanes and herbal remedies.

A modern dietician, Dr. Benjamin Feingold, has developed a system of diet which he claims to be particularly valuable in the treatment of children who are "hyperactive" and have behavioural problems, but which is much more generally applicable. The basis of his theory is that all foods containing synthetic colouring, flavouring or preservatives should be rigorously eliminated and also many drugs and artificial vitamin preparations as well as teas, coffee, pickles, vinegars and wines. However, he also considers that a large number of fruits and vegetables containing natural salicylates should be eliminated too, at least for a period of time. Many of the fruits and vegetables which are thus listed as salicylates are foods which have always been regarded as natural, wholesome and valuable and this leads one to wonder whether they should indeed be eliminated in the way suggested by Dr. Feingold and whether he has not failed to realize the great distinction which Lindlahr draws between the organic and inorganic forms of chemical substances. The former may do the body a great deal of good while the latter may do a lot of harm.

Some acid fruit may be taken before retiring. It is a good practice for everybody to have one meal of the day consisting entirely of juicy fruits or raw vegetable salads so as to give full sway to their purifying effects upon the system, undisturbed by other kinds of food.

Another fallacy of certain food reformers is the idea that acid fruits and vegetables should not be mixed at the same meal. Ever since we started in the sanatorium work we have mixed acid fruits and vegetables in the same salads with the best results. Many patients, who were impressed with the idea of the incompatibility of fruits and vegetables and horrified at the sight of our "mixed salads", were pleasantly surprised when they found that this "bugaboo" was only a matter of imagination.

It is impossible to make hard and fast general rules, as long as the human family is afflicted with so many varying digestive troubles. If all were normal, the normal diet outlined in Chapter I of this volume would do for all, with slight variations. But during the period of reconstruction and recovery from chronic digestive ailments, the diet will have to be adapted to individual requirements.

Coroborative Evidence of the Importance of the Positive Mineral Elements in the Vital Economy

The importance of positive alkaline mineral elements in the vital economy is indicated by the remarkable tonic effects of saline solutions on living animal and human tissues. Salts are compounds in which the hydrogen of acids has been replaced by positive mineral elements. These positive mineral elements are, therefore, present in all salts. It is now a well known fact that salt solutions injected into the rectum have a decided tonic effect, in cases of grave depression or suspended animation resulting from shock, great loss of blood, surgical operations, or other profound influences on the nervous system.

Saline solutions greatly stimulate the growth and activity of animal cells, even when detached from the parent organism. This is true not only of single cells, but also of entire organs, as has been determined by actual experiments. For instance, the hearts of frogs, rabbits and other laboratory animals will continue to beat when submerged in a saline solution, for a considerable length of time after they have been removed from the organism to which they belong. This seems to indicate a close relationship between the positive mineral elements contained in the salts and the activities of the life elements in animal and human bodies. These tonic effects of the salts of positive mineral elements explain why the latter have a positive effect upon the system, while the foods composed entirely of negative acid forming elements, produce negative effects.

110

APPENDIX I

KEY TO OUR SYSTEM OF RECIPE MARKING

We claim that we of the Nature Cure School have been able over the years to build up a science of Natural Dietetics and to reduce the problem of food selection and combination to an exact system. But most people, however understanding and well informed, find it difficult to apply the principles of Natural Dietetics in the kitchen. While they may fully understand the theory of food selection and combination, they do not know the chemical composition of the different food materials, and therefore find it impossible to select and combine to the best advantage. The same is true of physicians and students of dietetics. Though they may understand thoroughly how starches, fats, proteins and organic salts should be combined in order to meet the requirements of the body for the various elements of nutrition, they seldom have sufficient knowledge of food analysis to prescribe or carry out a system of rational food combination, such as taught, for instance, in Natural Dietetics. They would be at a loss to know in what proportion starches, proteins, organic salts, and so forth, are contained in wheat, beans, nuts, bananas, apples, or other food material, unless they had made a special study of food chemistry. Furthermore, the physician who possesses this knowledge cannot impart it to the nurse or cook who has to provide the food for the patient. The difficulty is increased in cases of sickness and invalidism, when special care in the proper selection and combination of food becomes a vital necessity, and when errors in diet may be far reaching in their harmful consequences.

In order to overcome these difficulties and perplexities of the physician, the nurse, the cook and the patient, in an easy and thoroughly practical way, we have evolved the following plan: we have divided all food materials into the following five groups:

Group   I—Starches
Group   II—Dextrins, Sugars
Group III—Fats, Oils
Group IV — Proteins: albumen, gluten, myosin, haemoglobin, and so forth.
Group   V — Positive Mineral Elements: potassium, sodium, iron, lime, magnesium, manganese and lithium.

Every recipe in a cook book, underneath its title, can be marked in such a way as to show the various food elements which it contains, in the order of their amount and importance. In order to simplify and to avoid confusion, we can use in these markings the initial letters of the food groups, (instead of the numbers of the groups), as follows:

St .... for Starches (Group I)
S .... for Sugars (Group II)
F .... for Fats (Group III)
P .... for Proteins (Group IV)
M .... for Mineral Elements (Group V)

For instance, if starches outweigh the other food elements in a recipe, St will be placed first and the other elements after, in the order of their importance in the recipe. If the organic mineral salts constitute the predominating food elements, M will have the first place. The food elements which are present in a recipe in considerable quantities can appear in black face type. Those which are present in negligible quantities can appear at the end of the line and be separated by a dash (—), in light face type. For instance, **St P** — F M.

In the following we give a few practical illustrations.

Combination Salad

Groups **M F**

Ingredients: Lettuce, cucumbers, tomatoes, Spanish onions, lemon juice, olive oil

Wash lettuce, removing defective leaves. Slice cucumbers, tomatoes and Spanish onions rather thin, arrange on the lettuce; serve with dressing made of two parts olive oil to one part lemon juice.

Lettuce, cucumbers, tomatoes and onions contain large quantities of the five positive mineral elements. Mineral elements are also predominant in the lemon juice of the dressing. The olive oil, on the other hand, contains nothing but various kinds of fats. Accordingly, this recipe is marked Groups **M F** (Group M, mineral elements; Group F, fats and oils). Both groups are present in considerable quantities, therefore both appear in black face type.

Health Bread

Groups **St P** — M F S

This bread contains about 40 per cent starches, 10 per cent protein (gluten), 5 per cent cereal fats and vegetable oil, 3 per cent sugar, which has been formed in the fermentation of the dough, and ten parts per thousand of positive mineral salts. Starch and protein, occurring in the largest amount, are placed first in the marking and appear in black face type. Fats, sugars and mineral elements being present in small amounts only, appear in the order named after the dash, in ordinary type.

Ingredients:

3 lb 100 per cent wholemeal flour.
2 oz fresh yeast or 1½ oz dried yeast
approx. 2 pints warm water.

2 large teaspoons honey.
1 dessertspoon salt (or less to taste).

In a small basin dissolve yeast with honey in a little warm water, which should be slightly warmer than tepid. Leave to froth up. Put flour with salt in large basin, make a well in the middle and add the yeast mixture. Gradually add the warm water, mixing with a spoon, until the dough is soft and elastic. Then knead with the hands, turning the bowl and folding over the dough, perhaps for about five minutes. Leave to rise in a warm place, covered with a cloth. Grease the tins and put to warm. After about half an hour — possibly longer — the dough should have risen in the bowl. Now knead again, which knocks out the air, and form into shapes to half fill the tins, kneading each portion on the table with flour to prevent sticking. If there is any dough over, this could be made into rolls using patty tins. Leave to rise again for about 15 minutes, then cook in the centre of a pre-heated oven, gas mark 7 (400 degrees) for about 20 minutes, then lower gas to 4 and cook a further 20 to 25 minutes. Turn on to wire tray to cool.

Notes:

If you prefer a quicker method, it is possible to produce an excellent loaf by reducing the kneading time and allowing the dough to rise in the tins, and then place straight in the oven.

For additional flavour, use ½ lb rye flour and reduce the wholemeal flour accordingly.

To increase keeping time, add 2 tablespoons oil with the yeast mixture.

Milk

Groups M S F P

In explanation of this formula, we will give the contents of milk in round figures. There is no starch in the milk. The starches of the ingested food materials through the processes of digestion have been changed into dextrin and sugar.

Group II   Carbohydrates, (sugars) — milk-sugar, 6 per cent
Group III   Hydrocarbons — Fats, 4 per cent
Group IV   Proteins — casein, 3½ per cent

113

Group V Positive Mineral Elements — potassium, iron, sodium, lime, magnesium, altogether 23 parts per thousand.

The Mineral group is placed first in the marking because milk is a positive food, that is, the milk is rich in the positive mineral elements in comparison to the negative food elements of the first four groups.

In studying these percentages one must not become confused by the fact that the mineral elements are present only in minute quantities, in parts per thousand, while the other food elements occur in much larger quantities in parts per hundred. The positive mineral elements, though occurring in food and in human and animal bodies in small quantities only, are nevertheless of immense importance in the vital economy of the body. They are therefore given first rank in the markings of the recipes whenever they occur in similar or higher proportions to those in milk. Milk aside from red (arterial) blood of animals is the only normal or standard food combination and therefore is our yardstick in measuring and estimating the chemical composition of other food combinations.

What Constitutes a Natural Diet?

Doctors and laymen who are not acquainted with the principles of natural dietetics ridicule the idea that it is possible to prescribe a diet which will "fit everybody". A careful study, however, of the explanatory articles in this volume will show that there must be a combination of food elements which, in certain well-defined proportions, will fit the demands of the normal human body. This combination must conform in its component elements to the chemical composition of milk or red (arterial) blood. In other words, any meal or diet, temporary or continuous, in order to be normal or natural, must conform in its chemical composition to that of milk or arterial blood. If we express this food combination in percentages of our food groups, the formula would read as follows:

A natural diet, which is to fill the demands of the human organism, must consist one-half of the food materials of Group V (mineral elements) and one-half of the food elements of Groups I, II, III and IV, (starches, sugars, fats and proteins). Any meal or diet composed in the foregoing proportions conforms to what we designate as normal or natural in food combinations.

Diet Prescriptions Made Easy for the Doctor

It will be seen that, no matter to what school of medicine a physician belongs or what may be his ideas as to the diet to be used in different diseases, the system here outlined will enable him to give his diet prescription in a few words, with absolute precision, covering every possibility of food selection and combination. Formerly, in a case of, say, Bright's disease, the doctor could only give very general directions. He would perhaps say to the patient: "Exclude from your diet all foods which are rich in protein, such as meat, eggs and gluten". But the patient or the nurse might not always know what foods are rich in protein, or whether a particular recipe contained protein in objectionable quantities. Furthermore, they might not know what to substitute for the foods containing protein so as to provide the patient with a variety of nourishing and appetizing dishes. Under the plan proposed in this book, the physician, if he desires to prescribe a low protein diet, rich in organic mineral salts, will write his diet prescriptions as follows:

R. Group: M — one half
St and S — one fourth
F — one fourth

If, on the other hand, the physician should, in a case of diabetes, wish to reduce the carbohydrate foods and increase those rich in protein, his prescription would read as follows:

R. Group: P — one half
F — one fourth
M — one fourth
Avoid St and S

As before stated, it is not possible to carry out these directions to the letter, that is, to exclude any of the five groups entirely. While most food materials predominate in the elements of one or two groups, they generally contain small amounts of the elements of the other groups in varying combinations. The latter appear in the markings in light face type. For instance, the substance of wheat consists almost entirely of starches and proteins, but it also contains fats and organic mineral salts in comparatively small quantities (starches, 65 per cent; proteins, 10 per cent; fats, 2 per cent; organic salts, 8 to 10 parts per thousand). The patient, or whoever is to carry out the doctor's directions in the kitchen, will always find it an easy matter to do so intelligently and consistently with the help of a cook book in which the recipes have been marked so as to show their predominant group or groups. All that needs to be done is to compare the diet prescription with the group markings of the recipes and to select those which conform most closely to the physician's prescription.

It will be seen that this system of marking all recipes allows the widest possible range of choice in the selection, combination and mode of preparation of foods. If there be restrictions in the use of certain food elements in certain diseases, as for instance, the exclusion of starchy food in intestinal indigestion, the group markings will indicate plainly and at a glance all those recipes which should be excluded and those which may be used in safety.

We have purposely allowed some latitude in the use of the dairy products, eggs, spices and condiments for the sake of those who may be in the stages of transition from a meat diet to the natural regimen, and also for the sake of those who do not care to apply the principles of vegetarianism to the fullest extent. Those who desire to carry out a vegetarian or raw food regimen more strictly and consistently may modify or exclude the use of dairy products, spices and condiments in the recipes to suit themselves.

A Timely Warning

This may be the place for a timely warning. Do not become finical or hypochondriacal over the matter of food selection and combination. The man who eats with a scale by his side, weighing every bite of food he takes, is to be pitied. His over-anxiety prevents the natural enjoyment of food, and tends to produce nervous and mental dyspepsia. It is not possible to conform exactly, by weight and measure, to prescriptions and group markings nor is it necessary in order to secure good results. What we are trying to supply (and what has been lacking heretofore) is a rational system of food classification which can be understood and applied by anyone possessed of ordinary intelligence in order to procure for himself or for those entrusted to his care, the diet which is most suitable for the individual conditions and requirements. If those who follow the general directions for food selection and combination given in this book will keep fairly close to the proportions indicated, they will always be within safe limits and need not worry about the fitness of their diet.

In cases of serious illness and digestive troubles, it is always best to consult a competent physician about dietetic as well as other treatment. It must also be remembered that even the most wholesome foods, in the best possible combinations, cannot be properly digested and assimilated if the digestive organs are in a sluggish, atrophic condition. In such cases these organs must be made more alive and active through natural methods of treatment.

APPENDIX II

UNCOOKED FOOD VERSUS COOKED FOOD

Much can and should be said in favour of raw or unfired food. Less boiling, roasting and fermenting, and more of raw food would undoubtedly do away with a great deal of weakness and disease. Nature did not create man with a cookstove by his side. Man existed on this planet for ages before he knew how to start a fire, and in those days of unfired food he was, undoubtedly, like all the rest of God's creatures who live in the freedom of nature, healthier and stronger physically than the present day diseased and degenerate product of artificial living and hypercivilisation. This does not mean that we advocate a return to savagery and barbarism, but we do claim that with the highest attainments of modern civilisation we can combine the simple and rational ways of living and of treating human ailments which will ensure health of body and mind, the highest efficiency, and the greatest possible capacity for the enjoyment of life.

The constant use of cooked, highly spiced and fermented food takes away the relish of natural uncooked food. It deprives man of the natural instinct and intuition for the right selection and combination of foods. The majority of people in this country, reared from infancy on the most unwholesome and haphazard food combinations, have lost the capacity for tasting and enjoying the delicate natural flavours of fruits, nuts and vegetables. Mankind, for ages, has lived almost entirely on cooked and highly seasoned foods and stimulants. This has atrophied the taste buds in the tongue and palate. Natural sensitiveness for the finest flavours of fruits, nuts and vegetables and other uncooked foods can be restored only by using the latter much more liberally in the daily dietary.

Fruits

The most delicious and wholesome raw foods are the juicy fruits. While they run low in starches, fats and proteins, they contain large amounts of the positive organic mineral salts (vitamins). They are, therefore, nature's own medicines — splendid tonics, natural stimulants, cholagogues, purifiers, antiseptics, anthelmintics and febrifuges.

117

The only medicines we ever prescribe in inflammatory, febrile diseases are acid fruit juices diluted in water.

The finest medicinal fruits are the acid and sub-acid varieties, such as lemons, oranges, limes, grapefruit, pineapples, tangerines, apricots, apples, greengages and other plums, and certain subacid varieties of cherries, pears, peaches, nectarines, and similar fruits. While these fruits contain highly organised acids, such as malic, oxalic and citric acid, they are very rich in the positive, alkaline mineral elements, and have, therefore, an acid binding and acid eliminating effect upon the system. The prevalent idea, encouraged by many physicians, that acid fruits and acid vegetables cause rheumatism and other acid diseases, is entirely without foundation. This mistaken idea has arisen from the fact that all juicy fruits and vegetables are rich in alkaline organic salts, which dissolve the acid deposits in the tissues and throw them into the circulation. This temporarily overloads the blood stream with acids in solution, irritating the tender membranes of the joints, muscles, brain and nerve tissues, and thus creating the various symptoms of collaemia or acute uric acid poisoning. As a result, the urine shows an increase in acids, xanthines, indican and other forms of systemic poisons, which, without an understanding of the cause of their appearance, are regarded as "deleterious effects of vegetarian and raw food diet".

This increased elimination is unavoidable, if the patient is ever to be cured of his chronic rheumatism and other acid diseases — yet fruits and vegetables are blamed for causing rheumatism.

Lemon Juice the Most Efficient Antiseptic

The fruit acids, instead of being injurious to the system, are powerful solvents for morbid accumulations of an alkaline nature. In the (external) treatment of wounds and bedsores, even of the most serious nature, we never use anything but lemon juice diluted in water — the juice of one-half lemon in a cup of boiled or filtered water. Lemon juice is a wholesome food and at the same time is the finest natural antiseptic in existence, while most of the medicinal antiseptics and germicides in existence are powerful protoplasmic poisons which benumb and kill, not only disease germs, bacteria and parasites, but also the healthy cells and tissues of the body. Since lemon juice is such an efficient antiseptic externally, it must have similar effects internally. This is true, not only of lemon juice, but also in a modified degree of all other acid and subacid fruits and vegetables.

Our treatment of wounds is, in other respects also, altogether contrary to the teachings of the orthodox medical schools. While they bury wounds under many layers of bandages, soaked in poisonous antiseptics, we expose them as much as possible to air and light. The results are

118

simply marvellous. Many wounds and sores which had entered upon the advanced stages of necrosis under the orthodox antiseptic treatment and old varicose ulcers of many years standing, we have healed perfectly with the simple lemon juice, air and light treatments. Some advanced doctors have even proved the truth of these statements during the late World War and have taken credit for a wonderful "discovery" and a remarkable achievement.

Fruit Juices the Best Medicines for Babies

All babies under our care, from the second week of their mundane existence, are given acid fruit juices in between the milk feeding. This is the best cure for rachitic diseases, because in the fruit juices the infant receives an abundant supply of the bone and tissue building materials. To give lime water, iron, sodium and other minerals in the inorganic mineral form, when the luscious fruits contain all these elements in the live, organic, vitamin combination is, to say the least, very shortsighted. The acid fruits also contain considerable amounts of fruit sugars — the finest form of organic sugar in nature.

Sweet Fruits

The sweet, alkaline fruits, such as figs, dates, grapes, persimmons, melons, canteloups, and certain varieties of peaches, pears and the like, are very rich in highly refined, organic sugars, all ready for assimilation, and contain considerable amounts of the positive, organic mineral salts. They are, therefore, nourishing, purifying and stimulating. Dates rank highest in sugar, but are comparatively poor in organic salts. Figs make a much better showing. While they contain in round figures 60 per cent of saccharin elements, they are also very rich in the positive organic salts, containing over ten parts per thousand of sodium, seven per thousand of lime, four per thousand of magnesium. This explains their excellent relaxing, laxative properties. Sweet grapes rank low in proteins, but high in sugar. They contain about one per cent nitrogenous elements, no fats, about 16 per cent of sugar, and rank fairly high in organic salts — about twenty parts per thousand. The value of the grape cure, like that of the milk cure, lies largely in the fact that it is a mild and pleasant form of protein and starch starvation. The grape sugars burn up (oxidize), and the alkaline mineral elements neutralize and eliminate the acid by-products of starch and protein digestion.[1]

[1]
The Grape Cure is a very valuable form of treatment. It was pioneered by Johanna Brandt whose book "The Grape Cure" was published by Benedict Lust Publications, New York, N.Y. 10016. A more recent book by Basil Shackleton, is published by Thorsens. Both these persons describe how they brought themselves back from the gates of death by means of the Grape Cure.

Berries

Berries are still richer in the positive, alkaline mineral elements than the acid and subacid fruits. Therefore, they possess great medicinal values. The country people of Germany gather, in their seasons, the different kinds of berries, and preserve and dry them for use in the winter. Bilberries, blueberries, blackberries, raspberries, strawberries, gooseberries, elderberries, currants and cranberries, besides being delicious raw foods, make excellent soups, drinks and desserts, and are to be classed among nature's finest remedies. They run from forty to one hundred parts per thousand in the positive alkaline mineral elements.

The widespread belief that the seeds of berries and fruits are responsible for many cases of appendicitis is another fairy tale. The best way to avoid appendicitis is to live largely on seed-containing fruits and berries, and on other kinds of raw food. The small seeds which are swallowed act as scourers of the intestinal tract. They stimulate the peristaltic movements of the bowels and are natural laxatives. Appendicitis, in ninety percent of all cases, is caused by a sluggish, atrophic condition of the intestine.

Bilberries, blueberries, blackberries are excellent medicines, not only for diarrhoea, but for all other ailments of the digestive tract. In severe diarrhoea, dysentery, bloody flux and cholera morbus, no food whatsoever should be taken — only water mixed with acid fruits or berry juice. Blackberries and raspberries make delicious drinks and are fine tonics for weak stomachs.

Nuts

Nuts are by far the richest foods in nature. They contain only about five per cent of water — all the rest of their substance is solid nourishment. On an average, they contain from ten to twenty percent of proteins, fifty to sixty-five percent of fats, five to ten percent of carbohydrates, and from ten to twenty parts per thousand of the positive mineral elements.

The most costly beefsteak contains only from twenty to thirty per cent of nourishing substance, and seventy percent of impure water. Nuts, on the other hand, are three times richer than meat in fats and proteins and their delicious flavours are best enjoyed when eaten raw. They are, therefore, the finest substitutes for meat in the diet of the vegetarian and fruitarian. The only danger lies in eating too many of them. They should be taken in moderate quantities only, and always in combination with foods of the mineral group. No wonder many people say "nuts do not agree with me", when they eat them by the handful after a heavy meal of meat, potatoes and vegetables. The vegetarian uses nuts, not with meat, but in place of meat.

120

Vegetables

The leafy, juicy vegetables which grow in and near the ground rank lower in proteins and starches and still higher in the positive mineral salts, than the fruits and berries. They are, therefore, best suited to balance in the diet the acid producing starches, sugars, fats and proteins. The mineral salts, contained in the juicy vegetables in larger amounts than in any other class of foods, are the real blood, bone and nerve builders, the most valuable antiseptics, blood purifiers and generators of the positive, electromagnetic energies of the body.

None of the vegetables belonging to Group Five, which are relished raw, are improved by cooking. The cooking more or less destroys the vitamins and dissipates to some extent the vital energies latent in the vegetable protoplasm.

Uncooked Cereals

Seeds are highly charged with the sex principle, which in physical matter is the highest expression of life force. All seeds, such as cereals, nuts and legumes, which can be used as foods, are, therefore, especially rich in the life elements — in vital magnetism or vitamins — and these vital energies remain unimpaired and most effective in uncooked foods. While the digestive apparatus, in the case of most people, through the constant use of cooked and highly spiced foods, has lost its ability thoroughly to digest and assimilate the raw starches of cereals, it is good practice to partake of some raw cereal at one or more meals every day. They should be freshly ground or cracked in the hand mill, or soaked, dried and flaked in a grain and nut flaker. Flaked and rolled grains can be bought in every well equipped grocery, but these seldom consist of the whole grains, usually having been robbed of the mineral elements. The surest way is to buy grains and prepare them at home. A mixture of rolled oats, wheat and rye in about equal proportions, with additions of pine nuts and raisins, makes an excellent and palatable substitute for baked bread. The flaked grains may be mixed according to individual taste and fancy, with various kinds of nuts, raisins, figs, dates, or other uncooked fruits and berries. A great variety of palatable and tempting uncooked food dishes can be prepared in this way.

Raw Sugars

Always the natural sugars should be used. Honey is the very best of all and should be given preference when available. Maple and pure cane syrup come next in order; then the brown, unrefined cane or beet sugar. The highly refined, inorganic sugars — granulated, pulverized and loaf—should not be used.

Food and Thirst

Those who adopt a vegetarian diet soon find that they are not as thirsty and do not require nearly as large an amount of fluids as they did under the meat diet. The juicy fruits and vegetables contain on an average about ninety percent water. These fruit and vegetable juices, prepared in nature's own laboratory, supply in the best possible form the demand for fluids in the animal and human body. They are cooling, refreshing, and saturated with the most valuable medicinal elements found in nature. These vegetarian foods, therefore, are non-heating and non-irritating, and contain in themselves large amounts of pure and wholesome fluids. Flesh foods, as we have learned, are saturated with uric acid, poisonous alkaloids and ptomaines, which have a stimulating, heating and irritating effect upon the system. This is further increased by the spices and condiments necessary to cover the unpleasant odour and taste of the flesh. Large amounts of fluids are required to counteract the heating and corroding effects of these systemic poisons, and to "wash" them out of the system. Herein lies the reason why a meat diet creates abnormal thirst and is most conducive to the forming of the drink habit, while the adoption of a fruit and vegetable diet is the best remedy for the abnormal craving for drugs, tobacco and spirituous liquors.

MEDICINAL VEGETABLES AND RECIPES

Carrots and Beets Good Worm Remedies

Carrots and beets are very rich in organic sugars and mineral salts, and are, therefore, excellent blood builders, purifiers and worm killers. They are valuable foods in all forms of anaemic and acid diseases. Children, especially those afflicted with intestinal parasites, should be allowed to eat all the raw carrots and beets they desire.

Pumpkin Seeds, Good Tapeworm Remedy

Peeled pumpkin seeds, administered after sufficient preparation by natural living, treatment and fasting, will harmlessly and promptly remove tapeworms, roundworms, pinworms and other parasites. This remedy should, however, be used under competent advice. Santonin, filixmas (male fern) and other poisonous anthelmintics may kill the worms, but they also paralyze the intestines — in many instances causing life long constipation and intestinal indigestion.

Flaxseed Tea for Colds

Flaxseed tea is a valuable remedy for colds, croup and catarrhal diseases. It has a soothing and healing effect upon the raw and sore membranes of the throat, and upon the digestive and urinary organs. Take a few tablespoonfuls of this tea when needed to allay the soreness in the throat and bronchi. The best way to prepare this is to boil a tablespoon of flaxseed in three cups of water for five minutes. Then strain and add some honey and lemon juice.

Rutabaga Syrup for Colds

Rutabagas (or Swede turnips) furnish another splendid remedy for croups and catarrhs. Take a large rutabaga, scrub clean with a vegetable brush but do not peel, then wipe dry. Remove top and scoop out centre, leaving a shell about an inch and a half in thickness. Fill cavity with unrefined brown sugar or with pure maple sugar. Now place in a very slow oven or on top of a cookstove for eight to twelve hours, in such a way that the sugar and the juice of the rutabaga forms a thick syrup. Care must be taken that the applied heat is not too great, lest it bake the root and dry up the syrup. If the sugar absorbs too fast, more must be added. A teaspoonful of this syrup should be taken whenever needed to ally the irritation and soreness in the throat and bronchi.

Kidney Tonics

Teas made from watercress, asparagus or juniper berries have a relaxing effect upon the urinary organs and are therefore valuable aids to promote the flow of scanty urine. Warm, relaxing sitz baths and hot compresses over the bladder are also valuable aids in relieving retention of urine. If the urinary organs are affected by inflammatory conditions, cooling compresses and sitz baths must be applied.

Onion and Grated Potato Poultices for Inflammation

Slightly fried onions make excellent drawing and soothing poultices for inflammations in the middle ear. Apply warm. Grated raw potatoes applied as poultices are the best of all remedies in the worst forms of inflammations of the eyes such as glaucoma, trachoma, gonorrheal infection and iritis. The raw potato poultices must be renewed before they become hot and dry.

Cottage Cheese and Gruel Poultices

Fresh cottage cheese or oat gruel poultices, warmed up to blood heat, are good ripening and drawing poultices for runabout abscesses, boils, furuncles, carbuncles and infected wounds.

Horseradish and Pineapple Good Counter-Irritants

Grated horseradish, pineapple or mustard make good drawing counter-irritant poultices for inflammation in the throat, lungs, or other organs of the body. The juice of pineapples (raw or cooked) is a good remedy for colds, coughs and croup.

Natural Laxatives

The best natural laxatives are figs, prunes and raisins, raw or stewed. In febrile conditions and when solid food cannot be taken, give the juices. Raisin juice acts better on some people than figs or prunes. Still others are aided greatly by eating young green onions, Spanish onions, scraped sweet apples, or by taking raw rhubarb juice.

Editor's Note

Lindlahr's aim in his writings and in his practice was to draw together all the "natural" methods of treatment so as to lay the foundation of a complete system of medicine or therapeutics. Dietetics, hydrotherapy, manual methods of various kinds, homoeopathy, exercises and a sound agriculture all had their parts to play. It is, however, remarkable that he did not have much to say about herbalism which is a very old traditional form of treatment in many communities in all parts of the world. There is no doubt that herbalism should form a part of Natural Therapeutics. It is true that herbs are used a great deal in the making of allopathic drugs and of homoeopathic remedies but this is very different from herbalism in its own right consisting of the use of herbs in their natural state. There are now individuals who practise herbalism with success and there are shops where herbal products are sold. There is a considerable amount of literature on the subject as, for example, "The Complete Book of Herbs and Spices" by Claire Loewenfeld and Philippa Black. As well as being used medicinally herbs have begun to be employed extensively in the making of cosmetics and ointments and in the care of the skin. This is much to be welcomed as it is becoming clear that much harm is being done by many of the commercial cosmetics now in common use.

APPENDIX IV

POPULAR SUPERSTITIONS

Strawberries and Cucumbers – Purifiers, not Poisons

Some writers on hygienic subjects have created a popular superstition that strawberries, cucumbers, tomatoes and other medicinal fruits and vegetables are poison foods, because they sometimes produce skin eruptions, diarrhoea and other forms of acute elimination.

Cucumbers as they come from the garden are medicine to the human body, especially in diarrhoeas and cholera morbus. They are homoeopathic to such conditions. It is wrong to soak them in salt, pepper and vinegar. In their natural state, they are great purifiers, counteracting the poisons of flesh foods, alcohol and tobacco. Because they eliminate the noxious accumulations of these poisons in a somewhat drastic manner, many physicians as well as the laity regard them as harmful and poisonous. This is "blaming the broom for raising the dust". When properly prepared, or rather when not prepared at all aside from cleaning, they rank among the most wholesome products of the soil. The rinds of the cucumbers contain a valuable kidney tonic and should not be removed if tender and palatable.

Grapefruit does not contain quinine, though like all other acid and subacid fruits and vegetables for reasons elsewhere explained, it is an excellent remedy in all inflammatory febrile diseases.

Tomatoes do not make cancer, but help to cure it. Most of our cancer patients, at one time or another while undergoing treatment, usually during the healing crises, develop a strong appetite for tomatoes, and we always encourage them to satisfy this craving to the fullest extent.

Lettuce is a splendid remedy for soothing tired and irritated nerves, and for relieving insomnia. Its sedative qualities, however, are not due to opium. Lettuce does not contain the slightest trace of opium, but it is very rich in the positive, alkaline mineral elements. These neutralize and eliminate the poisonous acids and alkaloids which irritate and over-stimulate the brain and nervous system, and cause all kinds of nervous troubles.

Peaches do not contain prussic acid. It is true that the seed of the peach contains minute quantities of this poison – not enough to be harmful – but the luscious flesh of the peach does not contain the slightest trace. It is regrettable that people should be frightened from enjoying one of nature's most delicious and wholesome products through this foolish superstition.

Watermelons do not cause malaria. That they do is a widespread superstitious belief among southern people, for whom plenty of fresh watermelons in their season would be the best possible preventive of malaria. True, watermelons in a condition of decay may, like all other such foods, become dangerous to health, but when ripe and fresh this delicious, juicy fruit is one of nature's finest cooling and purifying medicines – one of the best known cures for malaria and other febrile diseases peculiar to hot climates. If the southern people would use more watermelons and other juicy fruits during the hot season, instead of so much lard and other greasy foods, for which they seem to have a curious fancy, they would not be so prone to these maladies.

APPENDIX V

CLASSIFICATION OF RECIPES

In compiling his Cook Book, Lindlahr arranged the recipes under the following thirteen headings:

    (1)   Salads and Salad Dressings
    (2)   Relishes
    (3)   Soups
    (4)   Vegetables
    (5)   Cereal Foods
    (6)   Breads
    (7)   Rice, Macaroni and Spaghetti
    (8)   Dairy Products
    (9)   Eggs
  (10)   Roasts, Croquettes and Stews
  (11)   Sandwiches
  (12)   Beverages
  (13)   Desserts

He has something to say about each of these.

(1) Salads and Salad Dressings

The leafy, juicy vegetables and the fruits are most beneficial when eaten raw without dressing, or when prepared simply with lemon juice and olive oil. Never use vinegar or pepper and salt with lemon juice and olive oil. Lemon juice is the most delicious substitute for vinegar. Vinegar, a product of fermentation, is a powerful antiseptic and preservative. It is useful for preserving food in the pantry, but it is not advisable to preserve food in our stomachs. Vinegar retards digestion; lemon juice promotes it. An exception to this is the digestion of the starches in the stomach which is somewhat retarded by acid fruit and vegetable juices. Mayonnaise and French dressings should be prepared with lemon juice instead of vinegar. [1]

[1]
    Vinegar (acetic acid) is known to induce anaemia, haemorrhages, wasting and debility. Cider vinegar, however, contains ingredients which help to counter the acetic acid, and may be used in dressings. A teaspoonful each of honey and Cider Vinegar daily is considered to be effective against rheumatism. Cider Vinegar provides easily assimilated potassium which is frequently deficient in the average diet.

Every meal should contain a considerable proportion of uncooked fruits and vegetables, which are best served in the form of salads. In the summer, salads should take the place, to a large extent, of soups and cooked foods. For luncheon, an appetizing fruit or vegetable salad with whole bread and, if desired, a glass of milk or fruit juice, will be found fully satisfying and sufficient for the brain worker, as well as for one engaged in physical labour. The salad should be served at the beginning of the meal.

There are certain rules regarding the preparation of salads which should be observed in all circumstances. 1) Strong condiments and spices should not be used. They over-stimulate and thereby irritate the digestive organs, the nerves and the sex centres, interfere with proper digestion and assimilation, and thus result in a corresponding degree of weakness which affects the entire organism. 2) Lemon juice should be used instead of vinegar, for reasons previously stated. 3) Seasoning and dressing should be added at the last moment, just before serving.

Any of the following green vegetables may be served singly or in various combinations with suitable dressings, that is: lettuce is very appetizing with lemon juice and honey only, or with any good dressing; cucumbers may be sliced or chopped with a simple dressing. They are very palatable when quartered lengthwise and sprinkled with lemon juice and olive oil. Sliced onions, sliced tomatoes, cucumbers, endive, Swiss chard, young carrots, green peas in the pods, nasturtium leaves and green seed pods, celery, cabbage, young spinach, parsley, water cress and dandelions are good with different kinds of dressing, to suit individual taste. Water cress is very palatable with lemon juice and olive oil. The flavour of tomatoes blends well with mayonnaise.

For patients on a curative diet only the simpler dressings and salads should be used.

(2) Relishes

Tender raw vegetables make most acceptable relishes. Besides those most commonly used, such as radishes, onions, celery and ripe olives, we may use raw turnips sliced or grated, kohlrabi, carrots, artichokes or egg plant. Rhubarb makes a delicious and very wholesome relish. use the tender ribs of the leaves and the tender parts of the stalk, cut into small pieces and serve raw without any dressing. Raw cauliflower makes a palatable relish, the flowerets being separated and served without dressing; or they may be added to any of the salads, in season. Raw asparagus tips, or indeed the whole stalk when tender, will be found a pleasing addition to the list of available relishes, and may be used in salads as well. Raw sweet corn in the tender stage will be a surprise to those trying it for the first time. It may be served without dressing; or it may be combined with other ingredients.

(3) Soups

In the natural diet, we tolerate rather than recommend the use of soups. They are objectionable for several reasons. Most soups are not relished except when taken hot, and hot foods, especially liquids, have the effect of anaesthetizing, weakening and dilating the stomach. Moreover, like all other liquids, they dilute the digestive juices, all of which tends to weaken and retard the digestion of foods in the stomach. Soups should be taken slowly and as cool as they can be relished. It is well to take with the soup some solid food, such as whole grain bread, whole wheat croutons or Crispbread, or some vegetable relish, such as radishes, onions or celery. It is not at all necessary to begin every dinner with soup. It should not be served more than two or three times a week. The soup habit should be avoided.

Meat Soups

As far as meat soups are concerned, instead of containing the strength of the meat, as commonly supposed, they contain much of the uric acid and other morbid materials with which the animal carcass is saturated, and in addition to this, some fats and gelatin, but very little of the protein elements. The latter coagulate and remain in the meat fibre. Well informed physicians now admit that soups and meat extracts have more of a stimulating than a nourishing effect upon the system. This artificial stimulation is caused by the poisonous acids, alkaloids and ptomaines contained in the meat. The most valuable constituents of flesh foods, the animal life element or animal magnetism, is largely destroyed and dissipated by boiling.

Vegetable Soups

Pure vegetable soups, properly prepared, are rich in the mineral elements, which are of the greatest importance in the economy of the body, but care must be taken not to boil the vegetable soups longer than necessary, in order to avoid as much as possible the disintegration of the live organic combinations of the vegetable food elements and the dissipation of the vito-chemical life element (vitamins).

The foundation of vegetable soups is the stock made from leafy vegetables and roots, with a very small addition of peas and beans to supply the rich flavour of the protein which makes meat soups so palatable. Many forms of cream soup and thick soup can be made by the use of milk, flour and butter.

All vegetables may thus be utilized with the possible exception of the red beet, which would impart a reddish colour to the stock. The outer leaves of cabbage, spinach, lettuce, kale, the tops of beets and other roots, the tough portions of celery, asparagus and green onions, which usually go to waste, make excellent soup stock, because they are rich in the mineral salts – the essential element in good soup. To clarify the stock, use crushed egg-shells. The egg-shells should be washed, dried in the oven, crushed and kept in a covered jar until required.

Sweet Soups and Fruit Soups

Raspberries, blackberries, strawberries, elderberries, currants, Concord grapes and so forth, may be prepared, and served with dumplings.

Cherries and plums may either be rubbed through a colander, or, if pitted beforehand, cooked and served without straining.

Peaches, pears and apples may be cooked until soft and mashed through a coarse sieve.

Uncooked Soups

For those who wish to adhere to a strictly uncooked diet, there are recipes for soups made from vegetables and fruits without the use of fire in their preparation. It is possible to make combinations and have variety just as well as in cooked soups. Honey can be used in preference to the commercial sugar, because the latter is not an uncooked product. Furthermore, honey imparts a distinct flavour to the food which greatly improves it, It will also be found that by using vegetables in the uncooked state the desire for salt is greatly lessened.

Cooking Vessels

Fruits and vegetables containing acid are liable to form poisonous compounds with the metal in tin or copper vessels, or granite ware in which the enamel has been cracked. It is therefore advisable to use porcelain lined vessels. [2].

(4) Vegetables

Leafy and Juicy Vegetables

Leafy and juicy vegetables are the most valuable foods of the mineral

---

[2] Lindlahr was quite in favour of the use of aluminium cooking vessels, but since his time it has become well established that these are harmful, though it is probable that some aluminium alloys are less acted upon than others. Also, since his time stainless steel and many kinds of heat resistant glass and porcelain vessels have been developed and are readily available.

salts group (Group V). While the juicy acid and subacid fruits average from twenty to fifty parts per thousand of the positive mineral salts of iron, sodium, lime, magnesium and potassium, the non-starchy, leafy and juicy vegetables average from seventy to one hundred and fifty parts per thousand of these all-important, physiological and medicinal mineral elements. We have dilated upon the value of these positive, alkaline mineral elements as neutralizers and eliminators of poisonous acids and alkaloids, as blood, nerve and bone builders, as the principal ingredients in all the important secretions of the body, and as generators and conductors of electromagnetic energy. We called attention to the fact that the juices of fruits and vegetables, prepared in nature's own laboratory, supply in the best possible form the demands for fluid in the animal and human body. They are natural tonics, cholagogues and purifiers. They dilute and hold in solution the morbid, colloid (glue-like) products of starchy and protein digestion. The large amount of woody fibre (Cellulose) contained in the vegetables furnishes solid resistance to the intestines and thereby stimulates their peristaltic movements and makes very efficient scourers, purifiers and natural laxatives.

Richest in the positive mineral elements are cabbage, spinach, lettuce, watercress, savoy cabbage, endive, rose kale (Brussels sprouts), Scotch Kale, leek, celery and parsley. Next to these rank tomatoes, cucumbers, radishes, onions, horseradish, green peppers, asparagus and cauliflower. Splendid cooling and refreshing summer foods, rich in the purifying organic salts, are the watermelons, muskmelons, cantaloupes, pumpkins, squashes and other members of the melon family.

Roots and Tubers
For the qualities of roots and tubers, see Chapter XVIII, p. 88.

Legumes
The principal representatives of this class of foods are peas, beans and lentils. Fresh legumes in the green or milky stage should be classed under Group V. They contain considerable amounts of mineral elements and comparatively small amounts of starches and proteins. As the ripening process progresses, a large percentage of the mineral elements recedes into the leaves and stems, while the seeds themselves fill in with starchy and protein elements. Therefore, legumes in the ripe, dried state, such as beans, peas, lentils and so forth, should be classed under group IV. They are heating, flesh-building and acid forming. They are very rich in starches, but poor in mineral element, hence should be used very sparingly, if at all, in the curative diet; and in the

normal diet they must be combined with generous quantities of fruits and green vegetables, Used too freely, or without proper balance of eliminative fruits and vegetables, they may affect the health as dangerously as meats.

The Preparation and Cooking of Vegetables

Most vegetables and fruits are not improved by cooking. However, many diet reformers go to extremes when they claim that all or nearly all the organic mineral combinations in vegetables and fruits are rendered inorganic through cooking. This is an exaggeration. Cooking is merely a mechanical process of sub-division, not a chemical one, and mechanical processes of sub-division do not disorganise organic molecules to any great extent. However, it remains true that the fruits and vegetables mentioned under Group V are not improved by cooking. Only starchy vegetables and cereals are improved by cooking, and this is so because through ages of abuse our digestive organs have lost the power to digest and assimilate raw starch. The cooking serves to break up and separate the hard starch granules and to facilitate the penetration of the digestive juices.

As regards salt, this should be used very moderately, even by meat eaters. Its excessive use easily becomes a habit. Its elimination greatly irritates the kidneys and withdraws from the blood large quantities of serum. This creates thirst which necessitates the drinking of much water. This in turn dilutes the blood and other secretions of the organism, causing watery dysaemia of all the vital fluids. When the dietary contains liberal amounts of uncooked fruits and vegetables, very little or no salt will be needed. The addition of a little salt is permissible to vegetarian foods which contain large amounts of proteins, fats and starches, such as eggs, butter, peas, beans, potatoes, cereals and rice. Vegetables of the fifth group when properly steamed in their own juices so that none of their mineral constituents is wasted, do not need additional condiments. Their own salts are the best flavouring.

Steaming the Leafy Vegetables

After the vegetables have been thoroughly washed, drain them and place in a cooking vessel, the bottom of which has been brushed with oil to prevent sticking before the juices have been drawn out. In a few moments enough of the juices will have been extracted to cook the vegetable. Cook slowly till tender but not overdone, add a little butter, serving the juice with the vegetable. A little salt may be added in the beginning or while the vegetable is cooking. Cook all vegetables only as long as is required to make them soft enough for easy mastication, not until mushy. Overcooking not only renders the vegetable unpalatable, but dissipates to a large extent the life elements contained in the raw food.

If, as is the usual custom, the vegetables are boiled hard and for a long time in a large quantity of water, then drained, or what is worse still, pressed out, they have lost their nutritive and medicinal value. The mineral salts have vanished down the sink pipe, and the remains are insipid and indigestable and must be soaked in soup stock and seasoned with strong condiments to make them at all palatable. The natural flavours of the vegetables are the most delicious.

Asparagus and such root vegetables as carrots, parsnips and salsify should be covered with slightly salted boiling water and cooked gently, without covering, until the pieces can be pierced with a fork, but are not mushy. Drain, but do not throw away the water – use it for making soups or sauces. These vegetables are best served simply with butter. Beets are cooked in the same manner, in unsalted water, and the skins rubbed off when done. All these vegetables may be cooked in a steamer over boiling water if preferred. It will be found, however, that the green or savoury vegetables are of much better flavour if cooked in a vessel open to the air. The more nearly the regimen is confined to raw foods and the simpler forms of cooking and preparation the better will be the results. It should be noted that asparagus runs low in protein (2 per cent) and starches and sugars (2 percent), but high in the five positive mineral elements, about 50 per thousand. The tender stalks are delicious eaten raw by themselves, or in salad combinations with other vegetables[3].

(5) Cereal Foods

Cereal foods, on account of their great abundance, cheapness, keeping qualities and easy transportability, comprise by far the largest and most important part of human food. Some varieties of grains, corn, buckwheat or rice can be grown in almost any habitable locality on earth. However, grains and rice by themselves are not well balanced foods, as is shown in our tables of food analysis.

White Flour and Polished Rice
Cereals contain large quantities of gluten (from 8 to 12 percent)

[1]
Root vegetables may be chopped into cubes and cooked slowly in a little oil, with the lid on the pan, Leafy vegetables such as cabbage, cauliflower and Brussels sprouts need very little stock or water, and slow cooking in their own steam, just long enough to make them tender when pricked with a fork. Spinach contains so much water that it may be cooked without liquid, using only the moisture on the leaves after washing. Lindlahr deals further with the cooking of vegetables in Vol II, p 56.

which is equal in nourishing qualities to the protein of flesh foods. Furthermore, they contain from 1 to 2 percent of fats and from 65 to 75 percent of starchy food elements. The all important mineral elements, however, are represented in small quantities only, from 8 to 13 parts per thousand, and the larger part of these is lost in the refining process in the mill in order to comply with the fashionable demand for white flour and white rice. This foolish but almost universal custom necessitates not only the removal of the mineral salts which are located in and under the hulls, but also of a large proportion of the gluten, which is equal in nourishing value to meat; worst of all, it involves the loss of the vitamins.

The white flour and polished rice of commerce, having been robbed of their minerals in the milling process, contain only from 1 to 3 parts per thousand of mineral elements. Just think of the wasteful foolishness of this practice. The valuable gluten and mineral salts go into the bran and help to build up the healthy powerful bodies of our domestic animals, while man, the "Crown of Creation", grows dyspeptic, anaemic, thin and nervous on the white, starchy flour, robbed of its most important elements of nutrition. Furthermore, it is well to consider how this foolish practice contributes to the high cost of living; the protein gluten of the grains, which costs a few pence per pound, or less if ground at home, is discarded in the bran, and in place of it, meat protein, contaminated by all the morbid matter and systemic poisons of the animal carcass, is bought in the butcher's shop for about ten times as much.

Government investigation of the dreadful beri-beri disease, which since the American occupation has increased to an alarming extent in the Philippines and Hawaiian Islands, has revealed the fact that this disease is caused by the consumption of polished rice. When the patients suffering from this malady are given even small quantities of the "polishings" of the rice, which contain the vitamins of the cereal, they recover quickly.

While our "polished" white flour cannot alone be held directly responsible for such a serious disease as beri-beri, it is difficult to tell how much it has to do with the creation of the manifold ailments from which the civilized portion of humanity is suffering. Surely the discovery of the cause of beri-beri should be a strong warning against "polishing" our grains in a manner similar to the polishing of rice. We may safely assume that the great Wisdom which created this wonderful human body knows also how to feed it, and that, therefore, the safest way is to consume foods as nearly as possible in the forms in which they come from nature's hands. If a product has to pass

135

through the processes of cooking, spicing, fermenting and chemical treatment before it becomes edible and palatable, it is not a natural food.

The Structure and Chemical Properties of a Kernel of Wheat

To illustrate the fatal mistakes which are made in the production of superfine white flour and other artificial cereal food products, we give below a diagram of a wheat kernel, greatly enlarged.

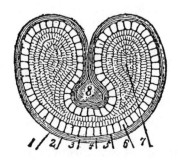

This illustration is taken from "The Foundation of all Reform" by Otto Carqué, an excellent little treatise on the diet question.

The outer layer (1) is the hull, or tough, outer coating, which, broken up into fine bran particles, furnishes necessary bulk in the digestive tract. The particles of ground hull in the whole grain meal act as a splendid stimulant to the peristaltic movements of the bowels. They also serve to keep the starchy constituents of the grain from forming lumpy masses in the digestive tract. They separate the starchy particles so that the digestive juices can better penetrate and digest the starch and protein mass. For these reasons whole grain bread and cereal preparations act as natural laxatives, while white bread and pastry made from white flour, together with meat, coffee, tea, strong spices and condiments are the most important causes of indigestion and constipation. What little the kernel of grain possesses of the all important positive mineral salts of iron, lime, sodium, potassium and magnesium are contained in and under the hull. The black, powdery deposit underneath the hull also contains mineral elements. It is the mineral salts which give tensile strength and toughness to the hulls of grains and to the protecting skins and rinds of fruits and vegetables; therefore, when tender and palatable, these outer coverings should always be eaten together with the inner, meaty parts of the foods.

Layers (2) and (3) contain nitrogenous matter and are rich in the alkaline mineral salts of silicon, phosphorus and potassium, which build bones and teeth.

In layers (4) and (5), we find a cerealine substance which gives colour and flavour to the kernel.

Layer (6) consists mostly of gluten, while the interior, white body (7) is made up principally of starch.

The germ (8) is the part which contains the life principle, and valuable, easily soluble organic salts. The germ also contains the natural ferments of the grain, which, under the influence of moisture and warmth in the soil, change the starchy and proteid materials into sugars and peptones, which serve as food for the growing stalk and roots in the manner that the substance of the egg serves as food for the growing chick. Diastase is the ferment which changes starch into dextrin and sugar, and peptase is the ferment which changes proteid into protose and peptones.

The germ (8) is the part which contains tne life principle, and valuable, easily soluble organic salts. The germ also contains the natural ferments of the grain, which, under the influence of moisture and warmth in the soil, change the starchy and protein materials into sugars and peptones, which serve as food for the growing stalk and roots in the manner that the substance of the egg serves as food for the growing chick. Diastase is the ferment which changes starch into dextrin and sugar, and peptase is the ferment which changes protein into protose and peptones.

able salts and ferments, are removed, leaving a product which has none of the most valuable constituents and finest qualities of the wheat kernel and which is therefore unfit for food. In the preparation of bread from such devitalized flour, the live organic mineral salts must be replaced by the inorganic table salt, and the organic ferments, diastase and peptase, must be replaced by yeast, soda, alum, cream of tartar or other harmful, mineral baking powders.

Bohemian Rye

The ordinary rye flour, the so-called bohemian rye, is made on the same principle as white flour, that is, much of the gluten, the hull, and the organic salts have been removed in the milling process. Furthermore, this brand of flour is frequently mixed with inferior white flour, which, on account of its dark colour, cannot be sold as such.

Rye meal

The rye meal from which the Germans prepare their dark rye bread,

if ground in an old-fashioned stone burr mill, contains all the constituents of the rye, and is, therefore, good material for our health bread.

Graham Flour
The original Graham flour, as advocated by Dr. Sylvester Graham,
was made of the entire wheat, but the Graham flour of commerce as
now sold is usually prepared by mixing bran with shorts.

Whole Wheat Flour
Many of the so-called whole wheat flours are not whole wheat in
fact. While they contain the starchy and glutenous parts of the cereals,
the hulls – and with them the mineral salts – have been removed in the
milling process under the mistaken idea that the hulls of cereals are too
coarse and irritating and therefore injurious to the digestive tract. This
is in line with much other "wisdom of the schools", which presume to
know better than mother nature what is good for beast and man.

Gluten Flour
From the viewpoint of our low protein diet, gluten flour and protose
are positively dangerous. They are the concentrated extracts of the
gluten or protein matter of grains, legumes and nuts. Gluten flour is
usually highly recommended to persons suffering from diabetes. We,
however, hold that a high protein diet is much more dangerous in
diabetes than a diet containing moderate amounts of starches and
sugars. Functional diabetes is caused largely by the clogging of the
capillary circulation with uric acid and other morbid materials produced in the digestion of protein food.

From what we have said, it becomes apparent why it is almost
impossible to buy in the open market a genuine whole grain flour or
meal. Practically the only way to obtain flour which contains all the
constituents of the grain is either to procure it from an old-fashioned
stone burr mill, or to grind it at home for daily use in a small hand
grain mill. [4]

Breakfast Foods.
With few exceptions, the widely advertised breakfast foods are denatured and demineralized in the manufacturing process. It is therefore
much wiser to use freshly ground or cracked grains. They not only

[4]
 Whatever may have been the case in Lindlahr's time there are nowadays a number of excellent 100
percent wholemeal flours on the market. It is important to buy stone ground flour as only by so doing
can one be sure that the whole grain, including the germ, is included.

make the best breads, but also delicious mushes and gruels. The hulls of oats, being very coarse and tough, must be removed, The hulled oats can be bought in the market as "grouts". Of the many cereal and breakfast foods on the market, those are best which are made of the whole of the grain, such as shredded wheat biscuit. We avoid the use of pre-digested and denatured foods.

Muesli is a popular breakfast food and can be purchased ready-made or may be made up from ingredients at home. This may consist of wheat flakes, oat flakes, rye flakes, sesame seed, sunflower seed, wheat germ and bran, and dried fruit. If desired, this can be soaked to make it more easily digestible.

(6) Breads

A good whole grain bread is the very foundation of a rational vegetarian diet. We soon realized this when we first tried to live on a vegetarian diet, and when we entered upon sanatorium work. However, we found that all the popular brands of flour and the various kinds of bread made from them, whatever they claimed to be, were lacking in some important constituents or were not as palatable and digestible as we desired. We then proceeded to try to combine the best qualities of different kinds of flours and meals into one perfect palatable and wholesome bread, and we believe that we have succeeded in producing something which has satisfied all demands as to pleasantness of flavour and perfect digestibility. In making our bread, we have wandered from the straight and narrow path of Simon pure vegetarianism to such an extent as to leaven our bread with real yeast or with some of the sponge of the last baking. Our recipe, (see page 112), makes the best of all health breads. The whole grain wheaten and rye meals should be stone ground. The addition of a little rye meal imparts a sweet, rich flavour which cannot be obtained from any other kind of grain. The worst dyspeptics seem to digest and assimilate this bread better than any other. Americans, who have never been accustomed to coarse, dark bread, almost without exception like it and soon cannot do without it.

The use of soda and baking powder in the making of breads, scones, muffins, etc. should be avoided as far as possible as it is not good for the stomachs and digestion of most people and can produce serious trouble if continuous or frequent.

(7) Rice, Macaroni and Spaghetti

Upon the proper cooking of rice depends its food value and its digestibility. The natural unpolished rice should be used instead of the polished and artificially bleached product. Unpolished rice contains only about seven parts per thousand of the positive mineral elements. The polished rice has been robbed almost entirely of its mineral elements and of the vitamins and fat. Natural rice requires a little longer cooking. It has a delightful nutty flavour entirely lacking in the polished rice and when cooked looks oily as if butter has been added. Wholemeal macaroni and spaghetti can now be obtained from health stores.

(8) Dairy Products

There is something in animal food which we cannot secure from purely vegetable food – and that is the animal (magnetic) life element, or, as we usually call it, animal magnetism. Each kingdom in nature is animated and controlled by a higher form, or element, of the great life force. This aspect of the diet question, which is entirely left out of consideration by most of our vegetarian friends, is fully treated in this volume. However, in order to secure the benefit of the animal magnetism contained in animal foods, we do not have to eat meat contaminated with all the impurities of the animal carcass. We can secure all we need of this animal life element in the dairy products in the purest and best possible form. Flesh foods we have to boil, bake, fry or spice heavily in order to disguise the unpleasant taste and odour of the dead flesh, and thereby much of the animal magnetism is lost. All the dairy products we can eat raw and in that way derive the full benefit of the animal magnetism which they contain. Therefore the liberal use of the dairy products is of especial importance in the case of weak, negative persons who have become so depleted in nerve force that they are not able to liberate and generate their own animal magnetism in sufficient quantities.

Milk

Milk is the one perfectly normal and therefore standard food in nature. It contains all the elements in exactly the right proportions which the newborn and growing animal needs for all the requirements of its rapidly developing body. These statements frequently bring forth the question: "Why then not live on milk entirely?" We have answered this question in Volume II, *Practice of Natural Therapeutics*, and have therein outlined a milk and fruit diet which we have found most beneficial in our work.

Buttermilk

Buttermilk is an excellent food for those with whom it agrees. In many instances, a straight buttermilk diet for a certain period will prove very beneficial. This is especially true in all forms of uric acid diseases.

Sour Milk or Sumik

Sour milk or clabber also has excellent medicinal qualities, and may be taken freely by those with whom it agrees. Sour milk prepared in the following manner can be taken by many who cannot digest milk or buttermilk. Let the milk, with full cream, stand in a covered glass jar in the sun until it coagulates, but does not completely separate into curds and whey. Turn out into a bowl and whip with an egg beater until it is of a creamy consistency. Taken with a few dates this forms a most palatable and nourishing meal([5]).

Cream and Butter

Cream and butter contain only the fat of the milk which rises to the top on account of its comparative lightness. The valuable protein materials and mineral salts remain in the skimmed milk. The latter is therefore not to be despised for its food values. In fact, its medicinal values are very much greater than that of cream or butter. We often find that our patients digest the skim milk much better than the full milk. Butter is not improved by the large amount of inorganic salt which it usually contains. The large amount of colouring matter is also often detrimental to health. The best butter from a hygienic standpoint is the sweet, unsalted and uncoloured butter.

Baby Feeding

The practice of feeding babies on cream diluted with barley water mixed with inorganic lime water, baking soda, milk sugar or table salt is positively harmful and preposterous in the face of the fact that human or cow's milk contains all the elements of nutrition in exactly the right proportions, and the valuable mineral salts in the live organic form in which nature intends them to serve as foods for animals and human beings. The cream and barley water are practically devoid of

([5])
Yoghourt is the form in which sour milk is now generally used and recommended and it tends to have a beneficial effect on the intestinal flora. It should also be noted that many people, especially children with allergy problems, find goat's milk more digestible than cow's milk and goat's milk yoghourt is often recommended. Lindlahr, though he considered milk to be a complete and standard food, containing all elements required in the right proportions, at least for growing children, did not believe in an entire diet of milk for therapeutic purposes except in certain special circumstances. He discusses milk diets in Volume II, Practice of Natural Therapeutics. The use of milk to any great extent is now rendered more difficult and unsatisfactory because it is almost impossible to obtain fresh cow's milk which has not been pasteurized and/or processed in various ways.

these all important mineral elements, and the inorganic substitutes act as poisons to the system rather than as wholesome foods.

For the foregoing reasons good cow's milk is the only natural substitute for human milk. Our analyses show that the difference in composition between cow's milk and human milk is not enough to affect the infant. The danger lies not so much in overfeeding on "rich" cow's milk as in underfeeding on watered milk and cereal dilutions and in poisoning the infant body with inorganic minerals. If, however, undiluted milk proves too rich, grain water may be added. In order to prepare this, take clean grain as it comes from the field, crush it in a new coffee mill, take three tablespoons of the crushed grain to one pint of cold water, heat and boil for one hour. While the gruel is boiling add enough water to allow for evaporation and absorption, then strain and add to milk one part of this grain extract to two parts of milk. Change these proportions if necessary.

When a baby is constipated, add extract made from oats, and frequently cool the bowels with cold water applications. This will cure the most stubborn constipation. If the bowels are too loose, add extract made from barley or wheat. Fruit juices and scraped raw apple are the finest baby medicines. They increase the supply of organic salts for blood, nerve and bone building and for purposes of elimination. During the first two months give one teaspoonful of orange juice, grapefruit juice or scraped apple one hour before or after each nursing. After the second month gradually increase the amounts of fruit. (See also Volume II, *Practice of Natural Therapeutics*, Part IV).

Cheese

Cheese is a very concentrated food. If made from full milk it contains the protein, fat and sugar of the milk and if made from skimmed milk (cottage cheese) it contains only the protein and sugar, but all kinds of cheese have been robbed of the larger part of the organic mineral salts. These are extracted from the curds by the withdrawal of the whey. This makes cheese a very unbalanced food, too rich in proteins, fats and sugars, and in proportion altogether too poor in the organic mineral salts. The compactness of the cheese interferes with its solubility and with the penetration of the digestive juices. Furthermore, the casein has been rendered less digestible through the cooking of the cheese. This explains why cheese is a "heavy" food, hard to digest and assimilate and why for so many people it is constipating. The processes of fermentation and decay which many kinds of cheese undergo before they are ready for consumption are not at all appetizing or conducive to good health. Cottage cheese in these respects is far superior to the more expensive, highly spiced and fermented brands. It is more easily digested because it has not been subjected to the cooking process, and is not as sticky and compact. Cooking coagulates and solidifies the albumen of the milk in similar manner as the white of egg. All protein foods, including meats, are therefore rendered less digestible by cooking.

(9) Eggs

Many people when they give up the use of meat seem to think that they must eat a great many eggs in place of it. Others eat large quantities of peas, beans, cheese or other heavy protein foods, in order to make good for the loss of the "nourishing" meat. This, however, is a mistake. The system may become saturated with poisonous acids, alkaloids by the excessive consumption of vegetable protein as well as by meat eating. Eggs also contain considerable quantities of uric acid, in the ready made form – it is claimed about five grains to the pound. The white of egg is almost pure albumen, which is a form of protein material. The yolk contains large amounts of fats and various combinations of phosphorus and sulphur. The last named elements tend to create, during the process of digestion, considerable quantities of sulphurous acid, an ill-smelling gas, identical with ordinary sewer gas; also sulphuric acid, commonly called vitriol; phosphorus and phosphoric acid; all of which, if they accumulate in the system, may become very harmful or destructive to the organism.

In view of these facts, it seems preposterous to stuff consumptive and other invalids suffering from "wasting" diseases, with enormous quantities of eggs, which their weak digestions cannot digest and which are bound to decay in their digestive organs and to fill the system with poisonous acids, gases and alkaloids of putrefaction. These patients cannot properly digest and assimilate a few eggs a day – if they could they would not waste away so rapidly. What then is the use of overloading their weak digestive organs with enormous quantities of indigestible ballast.

However, in moderate quantities, white of egg is a most valuable invalid food. When the powers of digestion are at their lowest ebb, raw white of egg, fluid or beaten, with or without fruit juices, is usually more easily digested and assimilated than any other kind of food. Also, eggs are of great nutritive value when eaten raw, soft boiled, or poached. Prolonged boiling or frying coagulates the albumen, making it hard and therefore less digestible.

(10) Roasts, Croquettes and Stews

Roasts and croquettes prepared from protein and starchy foods, such

143

as roots, tubers, pulses, cereals and nuts, mixed with vegetables and fruits, in the vegetarian diet take the place of meateater's steaks, chops and roasts. Many vegetarian recipes closely resemble meats in appearance and in taste as well as in similarity of elements of nutrition. The nut dishes may be too heavy for people with weak digestions, and we do not recommend them for everyday diet, but they furnish a pleasing variety for occasional use. Since pulses and nuts enter largely into these combinations it may be well to discuss briefly here the qualities of these foods, in order that recipes may be used understandingly.

Leguminous Foods

The principal representatives of this class of foods are peas, beans and lentils. They are also called pulses. These foods are exceedingly rich in protein and starchy materials. While the costliest beefsteak contains from 70 to 75 percent of water and very unclean water at that, the pulses contain only about 10 percent water, with all the rest solid nourishment. While meat contains about 20 percent protein, the pulses contain from 20 to 25 percent protein and in addition to that, from 50 to 54 percent of starches. It is the very richness of these foods in the negative, acid forming protein and starchy elements, which with the cereals makes them, next to meat, the greatest of danger foods. The protein materials of the pulses are made up of six elements: carbon, oxygen, hydrogen, nitrogen, phosphorous and sulphur. In the digestion and other vital processes in the system, these food materials are broken down, and the elements composing them may form many kinds of poisonous acids, alkaloids and ptomaines. One the other hand, these foods are very poor in the acid binding and eliminating positive mineral elements. Almost all diseases arising in the human body are caused originally by the accumulation of these morbid materials mentioned above. The effect of these poisons has been described in *The Philosophy of Natural Therapeutics* and earlier in this volume.

Young peas and beans however, as long as they are in the pulpy, juicy stage, are low in protein and starchy materials, but rich in sugar and the positive alkaline mineral elements. As the ripening process continues, a great chemical change takes place – a considerable proportion of the mineral elements recede into the leaves and stalks of the plant, while the seed greatly increases in protein and starchy elements. Therefore, sweet, young, juicy peas and beans belong to Group V (mineral Group), while when ripe and hardened, they belong to Group I (starches) and IV (proteins). In view of the fact that the pulses and cereals possess about three times the amount of nourishing materials as meat, the popular belief in the extraordinary nourishing qualities of meat seems pure superstition.

As stated before, the danger in the cereals and leguminous foods lies in their being too rich in the protein and starchy elements. This becomes more apparent when we compare these food classes with our standard food – milk. We find that milk, which nature provides as food for the new born and growing animal, contains only 4 percent of protein and 50 to 54 percent of starches. Yet we would expect that the young and growing animal and human bodies need much more of the cell and tissue building protein than the full grown and completed adult body. The food of the calf after weaning, in natural surroundings, consists wholly of green vegetation.

On account of their great richness in the negative, acid forming protein and starchy materials, the pulses and cereals must always be combined with foods of the fifth (mineral) group, which are low in proteins and starches and run comparatively high in the positive mineral elements that neturalize and eliminate the poisonous acids and alkaloids produced by the negative acid forming foods. Do not use vinegar with the pulses; always use lemon juice when an acid flavour is desired. The latter is rich in the positive mineral elements while vinegar is entirely devoid of them, and being a strong antiseptic it retards the digestion of the already heavy pulses.

Nuts

Nuts are the richest of all foods. They contain only about 5 percent water, while the highly priced meats contain 70 to 75 percent water. Nuts contain about 17 percent of protein, many times more than nature's standard in milk (4 percent), and in addition to this from 50 to 75 percent of fat. For these reasons nuts should be used sparingly only, and always in connection with foods of the fifth group.

Considering the great richness of the nuts in proteins and fats, it is no wonder that people complain about "nuts not agreeing with them", especially when a large amount of them is eaten after a heavy meal of meats and other foods. In the natural diet nuts, pulses and cereals are used in place of meat, not with meat.

The coconut differs from other nuts in that it contains less fats and proteins and more organic salts. The meat of the coconut, together with its milk, comes nearer to the chemical composition of human milk than any food product in existence. Some vegetarians allow peanuts a prominent place in their diet. But this is a mistake, since peanuts contain a higher percentage of protein (33 percent), than almost any other article of food, and also considerable xanthines, which have the same deleterious effects upon the system as an excess of uric acid. Pignolia or pine nuts, though very rich in proteins and fats, seem to be more easily digested than most other nuts. We have always found them a most valuable food for people with weak digestion. A generous quantity of popcorn eaten with black walnuts or butternuts balances the large amount of fat in these nuts and so tends to prevent digestive trouble.

General Directions for making Croquettes

In mixing the ingredients have the mass firm enough to hold together, but not compact. The croquettes should be handled as little as possible in shaping. Large spoons may be used for this purpose. In order to provide a firm and well browned outer crust, the croquettes should be rolled first in sifted bread or cracker crumbs, then in beaten egg, then again in crumbs. These crumbs should preferably be from whole grain bread, which may be toasted brown and hard in the oven before rolling or grinding. Baking is better than frying. The usual method of preparing croquettes by dropping them into boiling oil or frying in a small quantity of fat in a skillet or pan usually makes the food soggy, indigestible and unpalatable. Even when the frying is done most carefully so that a minimum of oil is soaked in the greasy crust, the complexity of the mixture renders the croquette unwholesome and difficult of digestion for most people. The best way to cook croquettes or foods which are commonly fried is to bake or roast them. They are just as palatable and far more wholesome. Place the croquettes on a hot buttered or oiled gridiron, baking pan or dish and bake in a very hot oven for about fifteen minutes until nicely browned. If they do not brown well on top they may be turned.

(11) Sandwiches

Much importance should be attached to the making of nutritious and palatable sandwiches. This is because many people are workers in factories or offices and need to take with them a meal conforming to the regimen prescribed for them.

In making sandwiches, the whole grain bread is always preferable. It should be evenly and thinly sliced, and fresh sweet butter used. Care should be taken not only to make good food combinations, but to make them appeal to the eye as well. Lettuce, watercress, tender Swiss chard or spinach leaves are welcome additions to most combinations.

(12) Beverages

Among the ingredients which can be used in beverages are grains, (e.g. barley water), apples, lemons, oranges, and the juices of cherry, strawberry, cranberry, damson and pineapple.

(13) Desserts

The best and most wholesome desserts are the fresh subacid or sweet fruits, and these should always be served when possible. Especially valuable are the sweet berries, peaches and melons in season. These should be properly ripened so that they have their full content of natural sugar, and should require no additional sweetening. They should be served cold but not iced. The raw fruits are especially desirable in summer. In lieu of fresh fruit, stewed, baked, or plain canned fruits put up with little or no sugar and without preservatives of any kind may be served. If sweetening is necessary, a little honey, brown or maple sugar or maple syrup should be used. Very ripe persimmons, especially the large varieties, are valuable, delicious and satisfying food. Next in point of desirability are the sun-dried sweet fruits, such as figs, dates, raisins, prunes, and pears. They are better for use in the winter since they are heat producing.

The richer and more complicated desserts should not be used in the curative diet and seldom used in the normal diet. These more elaborate desserts containing appreciable quantities of starch, eggs and so forth, must be balanced by the omission of like elements from the rest of the meal, using a raw relish and a plain salad and omitting proper proportions of rice, bread, potatoes, nuts or eggs from the main part of the meal when starch and protein predominate in the dessert.

APPENDIX VI

SOME SAMPLE RECIPES AND MENUS

Lindlahr believed that a "natural" and healthy diet was the most important single factor in producing and maintaining health and that it was an easy matter to work out and to follow such a diet in a rational and scientific way. As he expresses it, "there must be a combination of food elements which in certain well defined proportions will fit the demands of the normal human body". He gave a number of definitions of natural food and natural diet and worked out a system by which all common foods can be classified in accordance with their chemical composition and their nutritional function in the body. In defining what is "natural" food he says it is that food which appeals to the senses of sight, taste and smell in the natural condition as it comes from nature's hands.

He gives a number of instructions for making up a "natural" diet.

"A rational vegetarian diet properly combined, consisting of dairy products, the positive vegetables and fruits and just enough of starchy and protein foods to supply the needs of the body for tissue building and fuel material, will be found sufficient to keep people in health and strength in the most trying circumstances. It is sufficient if a fair proportion, say one half, of a meal consists of raw food and the other of cooked food". To make use of his system of food classification he says that "a natural diet which is to fill the demands of the human organism must consist one half of the food materials of Group V (Mineral elements) and one half of the food elements of Groups, I, II, III and IV (starches, sugars, fats and proteins). Any meal or diet composed in those proportions conforms to what we designate as normal or natural in food combinations".

Another test of a diet being "natural" is that in its component elements it conforms to the chemical composition of milk or red (arterial) blood which should be regarded as standards of what the body requires in the right proportions. From this it will be seen that Lindlahr regards a good and healthy diet as being a matter of proportions and not a matter of amounts or of calories, nearly all diets now in common use having a sufficiency or too much of carbohydrates and proteins but an insufficiency of positive mineral elements. Since

Lindlahr's time the movement for diet reform has acquired a considerable momentum though it has not as yet invaded the medical profession or its dieticians to the extent which might be expected or is desirable. However, there are signs that a change is coming in dietetic thought and practice, much of it in line with Lindlahr's ideas. For instance, the importance of having a proportion of uncooked foods and foods which provide roughage and vitamins is now very generally recognized.

There is also beginning to be a realization of the dangers of additives, preservatives and colouring matters in foods, of the undesirability of the present enormous consumption of tea, coffee, alcoholic beverages, fats and meats and the harmfulness of denatured and refined sugar and flour. In this connection it is of interest to note that there is not very much difference between the kind of diet advocated by Lindlahr and that which is recommended by the McCarrison Society and set forth in Dr James Lambert Mount's book, "The Food and Health of Western Man." The sample recipes and menus which are given here are mostly derived from Dr Lindlahr's original Cook Book with a few additions from other sources. Most of the recipes are marked or classified in accordance with the plan set out in Appendix I, so that it is possible to see the elements or groups which they contain in the order of their amount and importance.

Salads and Salad Dressings

Salad Dressing with Onion Flavour   *Groups* **M F**

To $\frac{1}{2}$ cup of oil or cream add the juice of 1 lemon and a pinch of salt. Beat well, then add the juice of 1 large onion or 1 grated Spanish onion or finely chopped parsley.

Salad Dressing   *Groups* **M S**

Lemon or rhubarb juice and honey, 2 parts juice to 1 part honey.

Thousand Islands Salad Dressing   *Groups* **F – P M**

Beat smooth 1 raw egg and the yolk of 1 hardboiled egg; add slowly 1 cup olive oil, then 3 tablespoons chopped ripe olives; add salt and paprika to taste. When ready to serve, add 1 cup whipped cream. Serve at once on lettuce hearts.

Salads

Raw Asparagus Salad   *Groups* **M – F P St S**

Cut into short lengths tender asparagus stalks, arrange on lettuce leaves, and serve with lemon or rhubarb juice dressing.

Carrot Salad   *Groups* **M F P**

Grate raw carrots, mix with pine nuts or grated fresh coconut or sprinkle with ground almonds. Serve on lettuce leaves garnished with ripe olives. Place a section of lemon on each plate.

Celery Salad   *Groups* **M F P**

1 pint celery chopped or dried. Mix with thin mayonnaise or sour cream. Serve on lettuce garnished with ripe olives or sections of tomatoes. 1 cup chopped almonds or pine nuts may be added.

Raw Sweet Corn and Cauliflower Salad   *Groups* **M F S**

To 1 part sweet corn removed from the cob add an equal quantity of cauliflower, chopped, a small quantity of minced celery, parsley or cress, and serve with salad dressing.

Nasturtium Salad   *Groups* **M F**

Shred equal quantities of lettuce and nasturtium leaves, heap on a platter or individual plates, dot with nasturtium flowers. Serve with French dressing or nut butter dressing, sweetened with honey if desired.

Uncooked Soups

Cream of Apple   *Groups* **M F P S**

Grate 3 apples (do not remove parings), add 6 ounces flaked pine nuts or Spanish peanuts, flavour with cinnamon or nutmeg and sweeten with honey. Beat together until creamy. Add 1 quart hot (not boiling) water. Heat the bowls before serving, or place them in larger bowls containing hot water.

Cream of Cabbage   *Groups* **M F P**

Chop very fine enough crisp, tender cabbage leaves to make 2 cupfuls. Add 6 ounces flaked nuts and rub together with a wooden masher until thoroughly blended. Add 1 teaspoon ground caraway seed and a pinch of paprika. Let stand about 15 minutes. Stir into the mixture 1 tablespoon olive oil or peanut oil and 1 egg, well beaten together. Add 1 quart hot (not boiling) water. Serve in heated bowls.

Banana Soup   *Groups* **F P S St M**

Into 6 ounces flaked nuts (preferably pine nuts or Spanish nuts) stir the juice of 1 lemon. Let stand about 15 minutes. Add 4 ripe bananas, mashed with a fork, and 1 grated apple. Beat well together, flavour with cinnamon, nutmeg, aniseed or a pinch of ginger, as preferred; sweeten with honey. Add 1 quart hot water and serve in heated bowls.

Oatmeal Fruit Soup   *Groups* **M S St P F**

Stir together 3 pints fruit juice (which may be obtained by pressing grapes, juicy berries, cherries, peaches, apples, etc. through a fruit press or coarse moulinex grater, or by soaking dried prunes or peaches in water for 48 hours), ½ pint orange juice and 1 pint rolled oats or wheat. Let stand about 10 minutes. Add 2 tablespoons olive oil sweeten with honey as required, beat well, and serve.

Cooked Soups

Asparagus Soup   *Groups* **M – St S P**

Cut about 2 dozen stalks into small dice, cook slowly until tender, in enough water to prevent burning. Add hot vegetable stock to make 2 quarts. Beat together the yolks of 2 eggs and ½ cup cream; stir the soup into this, and serve at once.

Tomato Soup   *Groups* **M F – St S**

To 1 lb tomatoes cut into pieces (or a 16 oz tin of tomatoes) add ½ teaspoon brown sugar and 1 bay leaf. Cook in 1½ pints water about 30 minutes, strain, and reheat. When boiling, add 2 tablespoons flour blended with 2 tablespoons butter; let cook 10 minutes and season with celery salt. Instead of flour, 2 tablespoons rice may be used.

Cream of Chestnut   *Groups* **F P – S M St**

Scald and peel enough chestnuts to make 1 lb. Cook in 1 pint water until soft, then rub through a mouli grater. Add 1 pint hot milk, season, add butter, let cook 2 minutes, and serve.

Cream of Leek   *Groups* **M F – St**

Cut leeks into small pieces, cover with water, let simmer until tender then rub through a fine sieve, or pass through liquidiser. Heat 2 oz of butter; add 2 tablespoons of flour (for 1 quart leek stock) let butter and flour simmer, but not brown. Add a little of the hot stock and stir until smooth, then add to the soup, which should be of creamy consistency. Season to taste, and lastly add ½ cup of hot cream.

Lentil Soup   *Groups* **St P M – F**

Soak ½ lb of lentils over night. Cook with a bunch of parsley in water enough to cover well, for about 1 hour. Add 1 cup tomatoes, canned or fresh, 1 Spanish onion and 2 carrots, cut into dice. Rub through a sieve (or pass through a liquidiser) and reheat with water or stock sufficient to make 2 quarts of soup, Brown 2 teaspoons flour in an equal amout of butter and add to the boiling soup. Cook 5 minutes longer, season to taste, add more butter, and sprinkle with chopped parsley.

Vegetables

String beans and Tomatoes   *Groups* M F – St P S

String and break into pieces 1 lb of green beans and cook in a small quantity of water about 15 minutes; add 6 tomatoes, peeled and quartered, a lump of butter, a little sugar and salt to taste. Let cook until tender and thicken with flour with butter.

Brussels Sprouts with Rice   *Groups* M St F P

Pick over 1 lb Brussels Sprouts, cook slowly until tender in a little water, to which a dessertspoon of butter has been added. When ready to remove from heat, add juice of 1 lemon. Put into the centre of a heated dish in a border of freshly cooked rice. Brown an onion in butter and pour over the whole.

Sweet-Sour Cabbage   *Groups* M – F S

Cut cabbage fine, as for slaw, cook slowly until tender with very little water, the juice of 2 lemons, a generous knob of butter, a pinch of salt, and sugar to taste. A little aniseed may be added if desired.

Red Cabbage and Apple   *Groups* M – S F

To 1 head of finely cut red cabbage add 4 medium sized apples peeled and cut into quarter sections, the juice of 2 lemons, half cup sugar, a little salt, and a generous piece of butter. Cook until tender, then thicken with a little flour dissolved in water.

Stuffed Eggplant with Nut Sauce   *Groups* St S F P M

Boil eggplant (entire) for 15 minutes, then cut into two. When cool enough to handle scoop out the pulp, being careful not to break the skin. Mash the pulp, season, and add 2 tablespoons melted butter, 1 cup grated breadcrumbs, 1 well beaten egg, 1 teaspoon of onion juice and a pinch of salt. Mix well, fill the shells and bake until browned on top.

For the Nut Sauce, add finely chopped walnuts or pecans to any suitable sauce.

Stuffed Spanish Onions   *Groups* M St F

Peel 4 good sized Spanish onions, remove the centre of each onion and chop fine with 1 green pepper; add a pinch of salt, a little melted butter, and 1 cup boiled rice; fill the onion shells with this mixture, sprinkle with paprika, add 1 cup vegetable stock and bake in the oven until tender.

Baked Parsnips   *Groups* St S M F

Scrape and wash parsnips, cut in halves lengthwise, part boil in just enough slightly salted water to cover. When partly done remove to a buttered or oiled baking dish, pour over part of the water in which they were boiled, sprinkle over the top some fine whole grain bread and dot with butter. Bake until cooked, basting with some of the water in which the parsnips have been boiled. Brown on top before removing from oven.

Filled Green Peppers, boiled   *Groups* **M St P F**

Cut the tops from large green peppers, scoop out the seeds, scald in hot water 10 minutes; drain and fill with equal parts cold boiled rice, young green peas and tomatoes cut into dice, mixed together and seasoned to taste. Replace the tops, set on end in a saucepan in water about one inch deep to which a lump of butter has been added; cover closely and let steam until tender, about 30 minutes, adding more water if necessary. Serve with tomato sauce.

Potatoes and Apples   *Groups* **M St F – S P**

Peel and cut into slices 4 medium sized potatoes, cover with boiling water, and cook 10 minutes, then add an equal amount of apples, peeled, cored and cut in pieces. Boil until soft, mash well, add a pinch of salt and a generous piece of butter; reheat and serve with brown butter.

Baked Potatoes   *Groups* **St M – P**

This is the best of all methods for preparing potatoes. Select potatoes of an even size, scrub well with a vegetable brush, wipe dry and put in a fairly hot oven. Bake until they are soft to the touch. If the potatoes are not to be served at once, take each in a cloth, carefully press and work with the hands and put back in the oven to keep hot. If handled in this manner without breaking the skins, the potatoes keep fresh and mealy for half an hour to an hour after they are done.

Baked Salsify with Cheese   *Groups* **St S F P M**

Scrape and cook salsify; do not cut; cover the bottom of a baking dish with bread crumbs, next with salsify, then grated cheese; repeat until the dish is filled, then cover with milk and put a thick layer of cheese on top, bake 30 minutes in a hot oven; serve at once.

Soufflé of Spinach   *Groups* **M F P – St F P**

Clean and rinse thoroughly about 2 lbs spinach, cook with knob of butter in the water which remains on the spinach until it is soft, about 5 minutes; cut with a sharp knife in both directions. Melt small knob of butter, sift in $\frac{1}{2}$ oz flour, stir well blended and add $\frac{1}{4}$ pint of milk. When it boils, add 1 oz Parmesan cheese. Season to taste, add spinach, the well beaten yolks of 3 eggs, and lastly fold in carefully the whites of the eggs, beaten very stiff. Bake 20 minutes and serve at once.

Dandelion greens, mustard, lambs lettuce, young beet tops, may be prepared in the same manner as spinach.

Baked Pumpkin with Eggs   *Groups* **M P S**–St F

Boil or steam pumpkin, pared and cut into pieces, then mash through a colander, removing the tough fibres. Beat 2 eggs very lightly add 3 tablespoons milk or cream, 1 tablespoon melted butter, 1 teaspoon sugar, and a pinch of salt, lastly stirring in the pumpkin. Beat well together, put into a buttered baking dish, cover with bread crumbs, dot with butter, and bake in a quick oven about 20 minutes.

Tomato Sauce   *Groups* **M**–S St F

Cut up tomatoes to make 1 pint (or use canned tomatoes) and cook with 1 onion (chopped) about 10 minutes. Add 1 tablespoon flour blended with a knob of butter. Let boil a few minutes, add a pinch of salt. Strain if desired, or put through liquidiser.

Curry Sauce to serve with Vegetables   *Groups* **M F**–St S P

Melt large knob butter in a pan; stir into it 1 large onion sliced small; let simmer 7 to 8 minutes, then add 1 sour apple, chopped; stir for 3 to 4 minutes; add 1 cup good vegetable stock and cook gently for 5 minutes; add 1 cup milk in which 1 dessertspoon of curry powder has been stirred until smooth. Let all boil up at once, strain, season, and thicken with flour or butter.

Baked Corn Pudding   *Groups* **S M F P**

2 cups grated corn, 1 egg lightly beaten, a little melted butter and seasoning; mix with 1 cup milk, turn into buttered dish and bake until the egg is set.

Cereal Foods

Breakfast Muesli   *Groups* **M** St **P F**–S

Mix wheat flakes, oat flakes and rye flakes with any type of chopped nuts. Include sesame seed and sunflower seed if available. Toast in an oven for about 15 minutes, turning over once or twice, to dry out thoroughly. If a toasted flavour is preferred this could be left longer. Add chopped dates, raisins, dried figs, apricots. This may be soaked overnight in fruit juice, or taken dry with a little milk.

Lindlahr "Vitamine"   *Groups* **M** St **P F**–S

Mix ground wheat, sweet corn, hull-less barley, flaked rye, oatmeal or rolled wheat with an equal quantity of grated cocoanut or pignolias, peanuts, pecans, walnuts or almonds flaked; or use a combination of any of these nuts. Mix with raisins or with dried figs, dates or pears chopped. This should be eaten without cream, masticated and mixed well with saliva, when the blending of flavours will be thoroughly enjoyed.

As a variation in place of the raisins or other dried fruits, bananas, pears, apples or sweet plums may be cut into small pieces and placed over the top of the vitamine, or berries in season may be used, and $\frac{1}{2}$ to 1 teaspoonful of honey added if desired.

Breads

Bran Muffins   *Groups* **St P F S M**

1 cup wholemeal flour, 2 cups bran, 1 teaspoon baking powder, 2 tablespoons syrup, 1 well beaten egg, a little salt, with milk enough to make the batter soft. Beat together until well mixed. Bake 15 minutes.

Bran Bread   *Groups* **St P M S F**

Boil for 20 minutes 2 cups bran moistened with cold water. When lukewarm, add 2 cups white bread, $\frac{1}{4}$ cup molasses, 1 cup raisins, 2 tablespoons melted butter; mix, and stiffen with bran. Let rise, then put into pans. Let rise again and bake 1 hour.

See also Health Bread recipe given in Appendix 1.

Dairy Products

Welsh Rarebit   *Groups* **St P F**

The addition of soya flour makes the cooked cheese easier to digest, and is economical on cheese. Heat 1 dessertspoon oil in pan. Add 2 flat tablespoons soya flour. Stir, adding very little water to make a thin sauce. (It will not thicken like ordinary flour). When cooked add grated cheese and stir in. Spread on toast and grill to brown slightly.

English Monkey   *Groups* **F P – St M**

Soak 1 cup stale breadcrumbs in 1 cup milk; melt $\frac{1}{2}$ cup cheese and a lump of butter together, add breadcrumbs and 1 egg, lightly beaten. Season with salt, let cook about 3 minutes, and pour over hot buttered toast.

Eggs

Eggs and Tomatoes   *Groups* **M F P**

In 1 tablespoon oil heat 1 onion, minced fine, until soft. Add a 16 oz can of tomatoes (or fresh tomatoes); let stew slowly 30 minutes. When ready to serve drop eggs (as many as required) into the tomatoes, cover a few minutes until the eggs are set, then pour carefully into a heated dish, Serve at once.

Eggs and Cheese Cream
Groups **F P – M** St

Heat together 1 tablespoon of butter and 2 tablespoons grated cheese; when well blended, add 3 eggs, well beaten and seasoned; stir lightly until the eggs are set, but not hard, Serve on toast.

Fruit Omelet
Groups **M F P – St S**

Use apple sauce or stewed pears, peaches, plums, berries or raisins. To 1 pint of sauce add 1 tablespoon fresh butter, sugar to taste, and a little cinnamon or nutmeg if desired; when cold, add 4 well beaten eggs. Bake in a buttered pan until brown, and serve with wholemeal bread. Grated raw apples make a delicious omelet.

Roasts, Croquettes and Stews

Jambalaya
Groups **M St P – F**

Into a buttered baking dish put 1 cup of unpolished rice, 2 onions, 2 red sweet peppers, chopped fine; 1 tin tomatoes (or $\frac{1}{2}$ lb tomatoes) and 1 cup mushrooms, cut into dice; mix well, and season with salt and a little mace. Put bits of butter on top, pour 1 pint of water over the whole, and bake slowly about 2 hours, adding a little hot water from time to time, as required.

Lentil Soufflé
Groups **St P – M**

Make a thick lentil purée; to 1 cup of purée add the stiffly beaten whites of 2 eggs; bake in a moderate oven about $\frac{1}{2}$ hour; serve at once.

Nut and Cheese Roast
Groups **F P St S M**

Chop 1 onion fine, cook a few minutes in a knob of melted butter, add a little water, mix with 1 cup breadcrumbs, 1 cup grated cheese, and 1 cup chopped walnuts; add the juice of 1 lemon, 2 eggs well beaten. Season to taste and add more breadcrumbs if necessary; turn into a buttered baking dish and bake in a moderate oven. Serve with a white sauce.

Chestnut Pie
Groups **F P St – M**

Heat 2 onions, chopped fine, in butter until lightly browned; mix with blanched chestnuts, cut in halves and previously cooked in water enough to cover until soft. Season to taste, pour into a buttered baking dish lined with mashed potatoes, cover with a layer of potatoes, heat thoroughly in the oven, letting the top crust get nicely browned. This dish is delicious if served with cranberry sauce.

Lentil croquettes   *Groups* **St P M – F**

Mix well cooked lentils, 1 chopped Spanish onion, ½ grated nutmeg, ½ cup cream, pinch of salt, 2 eggs and breadcrumbs to make the right consistency; shape into croquettes and brown in the oven.

Unfired Nut Loaf   *Groups* **F P – St M S**

1 cup ground almonds, 2 tablespoons each walnuts and rolled oats, pounded together. Mix all, moisten with milk or cream, season with celery salt and a little paprika; pack into a mould and place in the refrigerator for one hour. Turn out, garnish with sprigs of parsley and serve with slices of lemon.

Sandwiches

Piquant sandwiches   *Groups* **St P F M**

2 cups mixed nuts, 2 onions, 1 cup olives, chopped fine. Mix with mayonnaise dressing.

Dried fruit sandwiches   *Groups* **St P S M – F**

1 cup each of raisins, dates, figs, prunes, dry or soaked, and 1 cup of nuts, chopped or ground fine make a good sandwich filling. If too dry to spread well, moisten with prune juice or lemon juice.

Peanut Butter sandwiches   *Groups* **St P F – M S**

Sandwiches with filling of plain peanut butter, thinned with cream, milk or water, and a pinch of salt, are easy to prepare. Lettuce, cress, or chard improve them. Or the peanut butter may be well spread with a layer of whole raisins, or ground or chopped raisins and nuts, lettuce, cress or chard.

Beverages

Bran Lemonade   *Groups* **M S**

To 1 quart water add ½ pint bran and let stand half an hour in a cool place; pour off water, to which add juice of 4 lemons and sweeten to taste.

Apple Drink   *Groups* **M S**

Cook 2 lb apples, cut in pieces, retaining skin and cores, with 3 pints water, until apples are tasteless; strain the liquid and use hot or cold, sweetened to taste. Prune, raisin and fig drinks may be made in the same manner.

Plum Drink   *Groups* **M S**

Put 4 parts plums to 1 part water and cook slowly until soft, then strain through a jelly bag. Add 1 cup sugar to 4 cups of juice, or vary to

157

taste; heat to boiling point, boil 2 minutes, then fill bottles, cork and when cold seal with melted paraffin.

Orange Egg-nog

Groups **M S F P**

For 2 glasses beat the whites of 2 eggs stiff with 2 teaspoons sugar, and the yolk of 1 egg with 2 teaspoons sugar. Mix lightly, add grated rind of 1 orange and the juice of 3 oranges. Serve very cold.

Chocolate Parfait

Groups **P S F M**

Whip the whites of 2 eggs very stiff. To these add 1 teaspoon fine cocoa and 1 tablespoon honey; put 1 large dessertspoon in each glass, fill two-thirds with cold milk, then fill in lightly the balance of the beaten egg. A dash of grated nutmeg is a delightful addition.

Desserts

Dates with cream

Groups **S F M – P**

Dates, figs and prunes may be used for many desserts. Wash and stone the dates, chop and serve with cream, or they may be steamed until very tender, cooled and served with or without cream. Figs and prunes, if very dry, should be soaked in a little water before serving raw.

Steamed Apples

Groups **M F S P**

Peel and core apples, steam until tender, sprinkle with brown sugar and set aside to cool. Serve with plain or whipped cream. Or, when ready to serve, fill with equal parts of chopped walnuts and dates, and cover with whipped cream.

Oranges with Cranberry sauce

Groups **M S F**

Slice sweet oranges, sprinkle with sugar, pour cranberry sauce over, and serve with whipped cream.

Peach Pudding

Groups **M S F P**

Peel and cut choice peaches in halves, remove stones and fill centres with macaroon crumbs; put a tablespoon whipped cream on each half and garnish in any preferred manner.

Prune Soufflé

Groups **M P S**

Mix well 12 large well soaked or cooked prunes, chopped fine and stoned, with the whites of 4 eggs, beaten until stiff; place in a well buttered baking dish, set in a pan of hot water and bake for 30 minutes.

Rice and Apples   *Groups* **St M F – S**

Cook 1 cup rice in 2 cups water, or half milk and water, adding a good knob of butter and a pinch of salt; when tender, spread a layer of rice in a buttered baking dish, cover with apple sauce, then another layer of rice, and so on until the dish is filled; bake in a slow oven. Serve with cream. Any other fruit may be substituted.

Grapes in Jelly   *Groups* **S M F**

Make a clear orange or lemon jelly; fill individual moulds to the height of about 1 inch; when hardened, place in each mould a small bunch of nice grapes, and fill the mould with jelly to nearly cover the grapes. When cold, garnish with grapes. Serve with cream.

Steamed Lemon Pudding   *Groups* **F P St S – M**

Cream together ½ cup each of butter and sugar; add 2 eggs, one at a time, beat well, and add 6 oz sifted breadcrumbs and the juice and the rind of 1 large lemon. Put into a buttered mould and steam 30 minutes.

Orange Soufflé   *Groups* **M F P S St**

To the juice and pulp of 3 oranges and the grated rind of 1, add 4 ounces of grated breadcrumbs; beat the yolks of 3 eggs with 2 tablespoons sugar and 1 cup milk; mix well with the oranges and breadcrumbs, stir in the beaten whites of the eggs, pour into a well buttered baking dish and bake for 20 minutes. Serve with fruit sauce or whipped cream.

MENUS

Three or four course menus can readily be made up from these or other similar recipes and can consist entirely of raw foods or of cooked and raw foods. For instance, there can be a course of soup or relishes followed by a salad and then by one or two other courses composed of cooked vegetables and/or an egg or cheese dish or a rice, spaghetti or roast dish. The meal can be ended with a dessert.

A DIETARY REGIMEN

Lindlahr's disciple, Daniel Mackinnon, has given us an outline of the kind of dietary regimen to be followed by the average person wishing to put Lindlahr's dietary ideas into practice and to eat "naturally". Some modification is no doubt necessary in certain cases or in disease conditions and, in particular, anyone wishing to secure or hasten the elimination of wastes from the body should cut down or omit pulses, cheese, cereals, spaghetti and nuts until the desired end has been achieved. In cases where a definite form of elimination, such as boils, skin eruptions or discharges, is taking place, but without fever, three meals a day consisting of fresh fruits and raw vegetable salads only may be indicated until the condition is cleared up.

(a) Immediately on rising squeeze the juice of half a lemon into a glass, fill up with cold water, stir, and sip down slowly. Add no sugar.

(b) **Breakfast.** To consist of salad, cereal. Milk and fruit. Salad to consist of lettuce on which is placed a substantial helping of raw fruit or raw vegetables which can be sliced, grated or shredded. Avoid the use of vinegar. A simple dressing of olive or other vegetable oil and lemon juice is best. Lettuce is important as containing both iron and sodium. Cereal must be some preparation of whole grains, raw or cooked. If cooked it should be poured into a bowl and allowed to firm a little. It should be eaten with half milk and half cream which it is best not to pour over the cereal but to put into a cup from which a little can be taken with each spoonful of the cereal. It is important that each mouthful should be well masticated to prepare the starch for digestion. If this is done no sugar, fruit or sweetening need be added. After the cereal a glass of buttermilk may be sipped down. A dessert of fruit in season can finish the meal. If dried fruits, which are very good natural laxatives, are to be used, the fruit can be put in a pan, boiling water poured over it, and be left covered over night. In the morning it can be cooked for five minutes and little or no sugar will then be needed, but brown sugar, honey or maple syrup may be used to sweeten rhubarb or cranberries as desired. Oranges, grapefruit, bananas, bread, tea or coffee should not be taken at this meal.

(c) At mid-morning and mid-afternoon an orange or grapefruit may be eaten or a drink of fruit juice taken.

(d) **Lunch** This may consist of salad, cooked vegetables, bread, milk and fruit. One or two slices of whole wheat bread may be eaten with the salad. The vegetables should be cooked in as little water as possible and just long enough to make them sufficiently tender. If a little salt is used in seasoning it should not be iodized salt. A glass of milk or buttermilk can be sipped during the meal which can be finished with a dessert, preferably of fruit.

(e) **Dinner** This is generally best for the heavy meal of the day to be taken after the work of the day is done, as this gives the stomach the opportunity to carry on the work of the digestion unhampered and with a good blood supply. Dinner should consist of salad, cooked vegetables, bread, milk and fruit. In making a cooked vegetable dish a good combination is one leafy green vegetable, one root vegetable and a baked or boiled potato with its jacket.

Peas and the various kinds of beans should be used somewhat sparingly, say three times a week, in lieu of root vegetables. Soft boiled or poached eggs can be used about four times a week at one of the meals instead of cereals or cooked vegetables. Cheese too should be used only in moderation, but cottage cheese and grated cheese are useful in salads. Nuts too are useful in salads or with fruit for dessert. Macaroni, spaghetti and roasts, croquettes and stews made with nuts, legumes, etc. are good occasionally instead of the usual vegetable dishes. The drinking of water at meals should be reduced to a minimum, but milk or buttermilk can be sipped during meals. Tea and coffee should be avoided but the desire for a warm drink can be met by cocoa, chocolate or by some tisane or cereal drink. Peppery condiments, pickles and hot sauces should be avoided. No meats, fish nor fowl are necessary, and pastries are best left alone.

REFERENCE INDEX

Acids — destructive effects, 24–28; uric a., 25.
Alcohol — drinking of, 5; in body, 103; in bread, 103; causes overeating, 108.
Alkalis — relaxing effects, 28–29.
Amino-acids — 20–23.
Amylase or Amylopsin — pancreatic ferment, 37.
Analytical Food Table — 84–85.
Anaemia — feeding of, 10; one cause of, 58; need of sodium, 79–80.
Anger — causes indigestion, 96.
Animal Starch or Glycogen — 19, 37.
Appendicitis — caused by diet, 88.
Appetite — false, 94; control of, 94; loss of, 97–98; aid to digestion, 104.
Arguments of the Antis — 3.
Arterial Blood — as a standard food, 32; properties of, 86.
Arteriosclerosis — caused by uric acid, 25.
Assimilation of Foods — 36–40.
Atom — constitution of, 76–77; attractions of, 79–80; determined by electrons, 77.
Auto-intoxication — 7, 29.
Auto-suggestion — 95–96.

Bacteria — not cause of disease, 67.
Bananas — in diet, 91.
Banting Cure — explanation of, 82.
Béchamp, Professor — discoverer of microzymes, 72–73.
Beriberi — cure of, 56; cause of, 45–46; prevention of, 58; experiments on animals, 58; foods producing b., 58–61; caused by lack of vitamin B, 67.
Berries — properties of, 89.
Bile — flow of, 38.
Blood — arterial, standard food, 32; properties of, 86.
Bowels — see under Constipation.
Bread — fermented, 102–3.
Breakfast Foods — unnatural, 33.
Bright's Disease — explanation of, 25.
Bulk — necessary in foods, 23–24.

Calcium — in body, 80.
Calculi — caused by uric acid, 25.
Calorie — basis of c. theory, 44; fallacy of, 56; high c. food diet, 57; number in certain foods, 84–85.
Cancer — of head, 3–4; caused by diet, 88.
Carbon dioxide — not vital energy, 14–16.
Catarrh — in intestines, 76; cause of, 108.

Cereals — hulls have vitamins, 53–54; refining process, 59, 92; properties of, 92.

Cheerfulness — aid to digestion, 96–97.

Chemical Elements — of foods, 35; in pure form, 72–73

Christian Science — ideas on diet, 6.

Chyle and Chyme — 36–38.

Coal — latent energy of, 13, 49; vegetable matter, 13.

Coffee — stimulating effect, 5; retards digestion, 107–8.

Combustion — a form of oxidation, 12.

Condensed Milk — as a food, 61.

Constipation — forms of, 28–29; from protein foods, 29–30; cured by natural methods, 76; result of American diet, 88; use of dry foods, 106.

Cooking — harmful effects of, 55–56; chemical action of, 73–74; *see* Appendix II.

Cornaro — prolonged life of, 98.

Corpse Poisons — 2; soil for germs, 28.

Crises, Healing — food cravings, 94–95.

Crown Prince Wilhelm — 57–59.

Daily Rations — early ideas of, 32–33.

Dairy Products — 22; daily use of, 50; contain vitamins, 66; advisability of, 92–93; eaten with fruits, 109.

Death — as a change, 47; after d., 52.

Diabetes — one cause of, 19; a d. diet prescription, 57.

Diagram — of digestive process, 39.

Diet — why we favour a vegetarian d., 1, 88; a strict vegetarian d., 92; ideal vegetarian d., 93; idiosyncracies of, 95; mono-diet and others, 103–5; early ideas of, 32–33.

Dietetics — popular idea of, 7; in a nutshell, 35; see also **Natural Dietetics**.

Digestion — of starches and sugars, 18–19, 37, 39; of fats and oils, 19–20, 37–38, 39; of proteins, 20, 38–39, 81–82; of organic minerals, 23; of meats and eggs, 27; processes of digestion, 36, 39; purpose of d., 39, 40; of raw foods, 56; psychology of d., 94; aided by fungi, 102–3; hindrance of d., 96, 104; during crises, 97–99.

Diseases — result of imbalance in the body, 6–7, 78; from waste accumulation, 9–10, 24–25; need for inflow of vital energy, 41; fasting for, 42, 97–98; haemophilia, 60–61; caused by lack of vitamins, 64; not caused by bacteria, 67; natural cure of, 93; need of certain foods, 94–95; febrile d., 97–98.

Dissipation — return to, 4; effects of, 98.

Distemper — cause of d. in horses, 25.

Distilled Water — injurious effects, 107.

Drinking — of water, 100; excessive water d., 106–7; of beverages, 5, 107–8.

Dyspepsia — from wrong eating, 7; mental d., 96–97.

Eggs — as a main article of diet, 82; properties of, 86–87; in tuberculosis, 86, 97.

Electricity — in all substances, 76–78.

Elements, Chemical — of foods, 35; in pure form, 72–73.

Elimination — of meat poisons, 1–2; cures cancer, 3–4; depends on mineral elements, 10–11; of systemic poisons, 28; in children, 34; of waste matter, 97; in sickness, 97–98.

Emotions — poison, 2–3; destructive effects, 96–97.
Energy — in coal and ice, 13–14, 50; in food, 13–14; potential e., 17; in flow of vital e., 17; expended during fasts, 43–44; stored in plants, 47–48.
Enterokinase — digestive ferment, 39.
Equilibrium — necessary for health, 27; in all nature, 78.
Eruptions, Skin — helped by yeast, 75; caused by strawberries, 89–90.

'Famishing World' — quotation from, 55.
Fasting — decline of energy, 11–12; necessity of f. in disease, 42–45, 97–99; in Ireland, 43–44.
Fats and Oils — function of, 19–20; as a laxative, 30; digestion of, 37–38; containing vitamins, 65.
Fat Soluble A. Vitamin — 65–67.
Fattening Animals — for slaughter, 2; use of salt, 100.
Fatty Degeneration — cause of, 80.
Fear-thoughts — in animals, 2–3; poison people, 6; hinder digestion, 96, 104 (*note*).
Ferments — digestive, 37–40.
Fermentation — succession of f., 50–51; in whole meal, 63.
Fertilizers — for mineral foods, 69–70; green f., 71; for strong plants, 101–2.
Fish — properties of, 87.
Fletcherizing — 103–4, 105.
Flushing — with water, 100; in constipation, 106, Dr Tilden's change, 109 (*note*).
Foods — necessity of natural combinations, 6–7, 94; selected by appetite, 7; chemically pure, 12–13, 14; functions of, 18, 35, 42; digestion of, 18; variety of, 23; positive and negative f., 23; polarity of, 23, 78; destructive effects, 23; Nature's provision, 31; cooling f., 31; in daily rations, 32; classes of, 35; high calorie f., 56–59; cereal f., 59; containing vitamins, 64; raw f., 56, 67; cravings, 94; analytical f. table 84–85; idiosyncracies, 95–96; amount of f. necessary, 98.
Food Groups — groups I to V, 18–24.
Fruits — properties of acid and sub-acid f., 90; for entire meal, 106, 110.
Functions — of foods, 18, 35, 42.
Funk, Dr — researches of, 46, 53, 54.

Haemophilia — in the south, 60–61.
Haig, Dr — on uric acid poisoning, 25.
Healing Crises — fasting for, 42, 97–98; food cravings, 94; a cleaning process, 94–95; action of digestive organs, 97–98.
Hensel, Julius — teachings of, 55, 69–70.
Hindhede, Dr — on Natural Dietetics, 89.
Honey — a natural food, 61.
Hoover, Herbert — belief in calorie, 56–57.
Huntley, Florence — named life elements, 45.
Hydrochloric Acid — action of, 38.

Ice — latent energy of, 13–14, 50.
Indigestion — caused by American diet, 88.
Invertase — intestinal ferment, 37.

Ion — unit of electricity, 51, 77.
Instinct — animal, 7; versus human reason, 8.
Irish Hunger Strikers — 43.
Iron — in the body, 79.

Kant — 53.

Lahman, Dr — analysis of milk, 33; teachings of, 55.
Laxatives — natural form of, 23–24.
Legumes — properties of, 91–92.
Life — more abundant, 41; see also Vitamins.
Life Elements — same as vitamins, nature of, 13–14, 46; in foods, first discovered by author, 46; Author's definition of, 46; classification of, 46; vitochemical, 55–56; 87; classification in foods, Chap XVIII.
Lipase — pancreatic ferment, 37–38.
Lithium — in body, 80.
Liver — for storage of food, 37.

Magnesium — in body, 80.
Malnutrition — 7, 28–29; in spite of a proper diet, 76; result of anxiety, 96–97.
Mastication — of starchy foods, 37; necessity of, 105–6; Fletcherizing, 105–6.
Matter — conception of, by Pythagoras, 52–53.
McCann, Alfred — quotation from, 55; suggestions of, 58.
Meals — missing of, 42; frequency of, 106; drinking with m., 107–8.
Meats — contain faeces of cells, 1; infected, 2; proof of injurious effects, 3–4; prevents cure, 4; losing taste for, 4–5; lacking in vitamins, 5–6; odour disagreeable, 8; digestion of, 27; ptomaines of, 27; constipating, 29; in special diet, 50, 93; deficient in minerals, 58–59; in Banting cure, 82; properties of, 87; fish, 87; m. substitutes, 91.
Mechanistic Theory — energy from foods, 44; sun energy, 48–49; chemical activities, 50–51.
Medicines — medicinal value of foods, 10–11; 90–91; positivity of m., 78.
Melons — purifiers, 91.
Mental Dyspepsia — 96–97.
Microzymes — 55–56; in fertilizers, 71–72; importance of, 72–73, discovery of, 73; secrete enzymes of digestion, 102.
Milk — effects of, 29–30; as a standard food, 32; chemical constituents of, 33–34; not perfect for adults, 33–34; digestion of, 39; vitamin value, 54; condensed m., 61; properties of, 86; taken with fruits, 109.
Mineral Elements — essential, 9; necessary for elimination, 10; for soil, 10–11, 69; in body, 33; relationship to vitamins, 53; in fruits and vegetables, 53–54, 99; aid to health, 79–81; in water, 107.
Mineral Fertilizers — use of, 69–70; green, 71.
Mixing — starches with acids, 108–9.
Mono-Diet — 103–5; when useful, 104–5.
Morbid Matter — prevents health, 76; throwing off, 97–98.

Nature — provides seasonable foods, 31.
Nature Cure — combination of all that's good; 44–45; curing constipation, 76; used by charlatans, 93.

Natural Dietetics — simplicity of, 8–9; in a nutshell, 35; results not immediate, 76; for delicate flavours, 102.
Natural Food — definition of, 8.
Natural Healing — 44–45; many aids, 76; methods, 93.
Nausea — in acute diseases, 97–98; from mono-diet, 104.
Normal Diet — according to certain authorities, 32.
Nuts — properties of, 91.

Obesity — 100.
Olive Oil — taken in excess, 30.
Olives — as food, 91.
Organic Matter — difference between organic life matter and simple colloid compounds, 71–73.
Organic Salts — 31; importance of, 33; in wild flesh, 66; in fish, 87; relation to vitamins, 66–67.
Overeating — for fattening animals, 2; weakening effects, 97; one meal a day, 106.
Oxidation — various processes of, 12.

Pancreas — as a regulator, 19.
Peelings — eating of, 61, 88, 58.
Pepsin — stomach ferment, 38–39.
Physician's Work — 51–52; advice for treatment, 104–5.
Pioneers — in Nature Cure, 55.
Plato — 53.
Poisons — emotions, 2; by overfeeding and accumulation of waste, 10; from starches, 37; from ordinary diet, 99.
Polarity — of foods, 23; 78–79; in various kingdoms of nature, 77–78, in regard to sex, 78; of medicines, 78.
Potatoes — value of, 88–89.
Potential Energy — 17.
Potassium — in the body, 81.
Powell, Dr Thomas — theory of vital force, 14–16.
Predigested Foods — 14; advertised ones, 33.
Proteins — functions of, 20; forms of, 20–24; poisons from 25–26; produce acids, 29, 81–82; constipating, 29–30; digestion of 38–39; p. starvation, 104–5.
Psychism — tensed or relaxed, 29; brought on by diet, 74–75; 93, 104–5.
Ptomaines — 1–2; poisonous, 27.
Ptyalin — starch ferment in saliva, 37.
Pyorrhoea — one cause of, 58, 68.
Pythagoras — teachings of, 52, 76.

Rations, Daily — early ideas of, 32.
Raw Foods — for entire diet, 48–49; easily digested, 56; aid to health, 56, 67; claims of extremists, 73–75; tends to psychism, 74–75; for a short time, 75; dangers of, 92–93; raw meat diet, 93.
Refining process — for cereals, 59; for sugars, 59–61; reasons for continuation, 62–63; removes vitamins, 92.
Relaxing effects — of foods, 28–31; *see* Tensing Effects.

Rest — after meals, 105–6.
Rheumatism — inflammatory, 4; caused by uric acid, 24–25.
Rice Diet — not natural, 92.
Rickets — cure of, 54.
Roots and Tubers — properties of, 88.

Salisbury — raw meat diet, 93.
Salt — for soil, 66–67, 70; salt or not to salt, 99–102; in cooking, 99; not visible in iris, 100; injurious, 100–101; fattening effect, 100; on raw food, 102; lacking in Africa, 102; tonic effects of, 110.
Schuessler — teachings of, 55; 'Tissue Foods', 72.
Science — religious side of, 40.
Scrofula — related to meat eating, 2, 3–4.
Scurvy and Scorbutus — causes of, 68; cure of, 100.
Seasons — food adapted to, 31.
Sex — unnatural stimulation in children, 1.
Sexes — attraction of, 78.
Skin eruptions — helped by yeast, 75–76; caused by strawberries, 89–90.
Smoking — 4.
Sodium — in the body, 79; if lacking in food, 81–82.
Soil — starved for minerals, 66, 101.
Soul — ideas of, 52–53.
Standard Foods — 32; properties of, 86; analytical table of, 84–85.
Starches — digestion of, 18–19, 39; mastication of, 37; stored in liver, 37; with acid fruits, 108–10.
Starches, Sugars, Fats and Proteins — overeating of, 9–10; not alone sufficient, 12–13; digestion of, 18, 39; by-products of, 23, 25, 27–28; relationship to disease, 26; as a vegetarian diet, 32; excessive use of, 33; chemically pure, 72–73, 78–79.
'Starving America' — 9, 11.
Steapsin — pancreatic ferment, 37–38.
Stimulants — meat and coffee, 1, 5–6; return to, 5; deprivation of, 7; spices and condiments, 8; useless without life, 42.
Strawberries — cause of rash, 89–90.
Substitutes — for old-fashioned foods, 60–61, for meats, 91.
Sugar — digestion of, 39; refined, 59–61; juices of s. cane, 60.
Sun Energy — in food, 48–49.
'Stuffing' — treatment of, 10, 97.

Tapeworms and Trichinae — in meat, 2; *see* Appendix III, 123.
Taste — destroyed by artificial stimulation, 8; of delicate flavours, 102.
Tea — damages digestion, 108.
Temperature — of the body, 11–12; during fasting, 43–44; heat necessary to keep up t., 44.
Tensing Effects — of foods, 28–31; *see* Relaxing Effects.
Thirst — caused by salt, 100; drinking at meals to satisfy t., 107–08.
Tilden, Dr — recantations of, 109 (*note*).
Tobacco — causes rheumatism, 4.
Trypsin – pancreatic ferment, 38–39.
Tuberculosis — overfeeding in, 10, 97; result of modern diet, 61; need of sodium, 80; use of eggs in, 86, 97.

Uric Acid — in meats, 1, 4; cause of disease, 24–25, 88; poisoning, 29; grape cure, 104–5.

Vegetables — rich in protein, 30; rich in organic salts, 31, 54; raised at Elmhurst, 70; properties of, 87; as a strict diet, 92.
Vegetarianism — ideas from German book, 47; Simon pure, 66.
Vital Energy — *see* Vital Force; during fasting, 11; true source of, 17.
Vital Force — source of, 11–13; Dr Powell's theory of, 14–16; animates atom and solar systems, 16; inflow of, 17, 40–41, 44–45; increase of, 41–42; decrease of, 42; source of (translation), 47–49; material conception of, 50; vital conception of, 51; source of, 51; *see* Vital Energy.
Vitamins — in meats, 5–6; related to amino acids, 21–22, meaning of, 45–46; early articles on, 45–49; minerals and v., 53–54; in cereal hulls and fruit rinds, 53–55; in fresh vegetables and milk, effect of processing, 61; table of, 64; name of, 65; effects of cooking, 73–75.

Water — distilled, 107; at meals, 107–8; Dr Tilden's change, 109 (*note*).
Water Soluble B Vitamin — 67.
Water Soluble C Vitamin — 68.
Whole Grain Products — 53–54; opposed by manufacturers, 61–62.
Wood Ash — for fertilizer, 70.
Woods – Hutchinson — on dietetics, 54.
Working Men — usual diet, 58.

X-rays — 76–77.

Yeast — as a medicine, 75–76; in digestion, 75; ordinary dose, 76, in bread, 75, 102–3.